Neuromuscular Disorders

Neuromuscular Disorders

A Symptoms and Signs Approach to Differential Diagnosis and Treatment

Editor

Nicholas J. Silvestri, MD
Associate Professor of Neurology
Department of Neurology
University at Buffalo Jacobs School of Medicine & Biomedical Sciences
Buffalo, New York

demosMEDICAL
An Imprint of Springer Publishing

Visit our website at www.springerpub.com

ISBN: 9780826171986
ebook ISBN: 9780826171993

Acquisitions Editor: Beth Barry
Compositor: Exeter Premedia Services Private Ltd.

Medicine is an ever-changing science. Research and clinical experience are continually
expanding our knowledge, in particular our understanding of proper treatment and
drug therapy. The authors, editors, and publisher have made every effort to ensure
that all information in this book is in accordance with the state of knowledge at the
time of production of the book. Nevertheless, the authors, editors, and publisher are
not responsible for errors or omissions or for any consequences from application of
the information in this book and make no warranty, expressed or implied, with respect
to the contents of the publication. Every reader should examine carefully the package
inserts accompanying each drug and should carefully check whether the dosage sched-
ules mentioned therein or the contraindications stated by the manufacturer differ from
the statements made in this book. Such examination is particularly important with
drugs that are either rarely used or have been newly released on the market.

Library of Congress Cataloging-in-Publication Data

Names: Silvestri, Nicholas J., editor.
Title: Neuromuscular disorders: a symptoms and signs approach to
  differential diagnosis and treatment / Nicholas J. Silvestri, editor.
Other titles: Neuromuscular disorders (Silvestri)
Description: New York: Demos Medical Publishing/Springer Publishing Company,
  [2018] | Includes bibliographical references and index.
Identifiers: LCCN 2017034196 | ISBN 9780826171986 | ISBN 9780826171993 (e-book)
Subjects: | MESH: Neuromuscular Diseases—diagnosis | Neuromuscular
  Diseases—therapy
Classification: LCC RC925.55 | NLM WE 550 | DDC 616.7/44—dc23
LC record available at https://lccn.loc.gov/2017034196

Printed in the United States of America by McNaughton & Gunn.
17 18 19 20 21 / 5 4 3 2 1

For my students, teachers, colleagues, and especially for my family

Contents

Contributors

Yaacov Anziska, MD, MS, Assistant Professor of Neurology, Department of Neurology, SUNY Downstate Medical Center, Brooklyn, New York

Carolina Barnett, MD, PhD, Assistant Professor, Division of Neurology, Department of Medicine, University Health Network, University of Toronto, Toronto, Ontario, Canada

Richard J. Barohn, MD, Gertrude and Dewey Ziegler Professor of Neurology, University Distinguished Professor, Vice Chancellor for Research, President, Research Institute, University of Kansas Medical Center, Kansas City, Kansas

Ari Breiner, MD, MSc, FRCPC, Assistant Professor, Division of Neurology, Department of Medicine, University Health Network, University of Toronto, Toronto, Ontario, Canada

Mazen M. Dimachkie, MD, Professor of Neurology, Director, Neuromuscular Division, Executive Vice Chairman and Vice Chairman for Research Programs, Department of Neurology, University of Kansas Medical Center, Kansas City, Kansas

Kelly G. Gwathmey, MD, Assistant Professor of Neurology, Department of Neurology, University of Virginia, Charlottesville, Virginia

Michael K. Hehir, MD, Associate Professor, Division Chief, Neuromuscular Medicine, Department of Neurosciences, Larner College of Medicine at the University of Vermont, Burlington, Vermont

Aaron Izenberg, MD, FRCPC, Division of Neurology, Department of Medicine, Sunnybrook Health Sciences Centre, University of Toronto, Toronto, Ontario, Canada

Nora Jovanovich, MD, Department of Neurology, University of Virginia, Charlottesville, Virginia

Charles Kassardjian, MD, FRCP, Division of Neurology, Department of Medicine, St. Michael's Hospital and University of Toronto, Toronto, Ontario, Canada

Hans D. Katzberg, MD, MSc, FRCPC, Associate Professor, Division of Neurology, Department of Medicine, University Health Network, University of Toronto, Toronto, Ontario, Canada

David Lacomis, MD, Professor of Neurology and Pathology; Chief, Division of Neuromuscular Diseases, Departments of Neurology and Pathology (Neuropathology), University of Pittsburgh School of Medicine, Pittsburgh, Pennsylvania

Diana Mnatsakanova, MD, Clinical Neurophysiology Fellow, Department of Neurology, University of Pittsburgh School of Medicine, Pittsburgh, Pennsylvania

Mamatha Pasnoor, MD, Associate Professor of Neurology, Program Director, Clinical Neurophysiology, Associate Program Director Neurology Residency Program, Associate Program Director Neuromuscular Medicine, University of Kansas Medical Center, Kansas City, Kansas

Karin Provost, DO, PhD, Assistant Professor of Medicine, Department of Internal Medicine, Pulmonary Division, University at Buffalo Jacobs School of Medicine & Biomedical Sciences, Buffalo, New York

Daniel W. Sheehan, PhD, MD, Associate Professor of Pediatrics, Department of Pediatrics, Pulmonary Division, University at Buffalo Jacobs School of Medicine & Biomedical Sciences, Buffalo, New York

Nicholas J. Silvestri, MD, Associate Professor of Neurology, Department of Neurology, University at Buffalo Jacobs School of Medicine & Biomedical Sciences, Buffalo, New York

Andrew W. Tarulli, MD, Department of Neurology, Atlantic Neuroscience Institute, Overlook Medical Center, Summit, New Jersey; Clinical Associate Professor, Sidney Kimmel Medical College of Thomas Jefferson University, Philadelphia, Pennsylvania

Simona Treidler, MD, Clinical Neurophysiology Fellow, Department of Neurology, SUNY Downstate Medical Center, Brooklyn, New York

Foreword

With *Neuromuscular Disorders: A Symptoms and Signs Approach to Differential Diagnosis and Treatment,* Nick Silvestri and his talented co-authors have created a novel and valuable resource for both neurologists and generalists. In contrast to the disease classification or diagnostic testing that provides an organizational framework for most texts on neuromuscular disorders, Silvestri and his colleagues have returned to the basics, framing the book around the initial interaction we have with patients—how and what are they feeling and what do we find on their neuromuscular examination.

Chapters of the book are divided into global presentations that should be familiar to neurologists and other healthcare providers. For instance, limb weakness is covered in separate chapters depending on whether the presentation is acute, subacute, or chronic. The topic of episodic weakness and exercise intolerance, perhaps less familiar to non-neuromuscular practitioners, merits its own chapter, as does ocular and bulbar weakness and respiratory dysfunction. There are two chapters that concentrate on sensory impairment and pain, and an initial chapter devoted to the interpretation of diagnostic testing.

Indeed, this text provides guidance well beyond the spectrum of neuromuscular disorders. Signs, for instance, are examined from the perspective of both central and peripheral nervous system causes, with etiologies succinctly outlined for quick review by the provider. Clinical pearls are offered to refine both history-taking and examination skills. Key features of neuromuscular disorders that present with the symptoms and signs discussed earlier in each chapter are summarized in tables, at times with guidance on laboratory testing to help narrow the differential diagnosis. Finally, there are brief overviews of treatment and management.

This granular approach, beginning with key elements from the history and physical examination, should be particularly useful for general neurologists and other practitioners who encounter neuromuscular disease outside of specialty, referral clinics. Its expanded sections that offer further detail, I believe, will be of use for neuromuscular medicine fellows and their faculty mentors. As I was reviewing it, I felt the book would make a wonderful companion to Aziz Shaibani's *A Video Atlas of Neuromuscular Disorders*, a video and photographic resource that likewise follows a symptoms and signs framework.

The pattern-recognition approach that courses through these recent works, of course, lies at the foundation of teaching neurology, whether the focus is neuromuscular disease or something else. But in this age of technological advances and ever more complex diagnostic techniques, such a foundation is often forgotten or taken for granted. It is refreshing to have this new neuromuscular textbook, which reminds us of the value and rationality of returning to the basics.

Gil I. Wolfe, MD
Irvin and Rosemary Smith Professor and Chairman,
Department of Neurology
Jacobs School of Medicine & Biomedical Sciences,
University at Buffalo/SUNY

Preface

The field of neuromuscular medicine has grown considerably even since I graduated from fellowship just a few years ago, with significant advances in diagnostic testing and treatment having emerged. While this book was being written, the first drugs were approved for Duchenne muscular dystrophy and spinal muscular atrophy, as was only the second drug in almost 20 years to treat amyotrophic lateral sclerosis. Laboratories around the world are working diligently to determine the causes of and treatments for these and many other neurologic disorders. In this context, it is now more important than ever to make firm and accurate diagnoses in our patients.

As asserted in each and every chapter of this book, the history and examination are of paramount importance to guide a rational workup leading to a diagnosis and directed treatment in the patients whom we care for. This was the rationale for writing *Neuromuscular Disorders: A Symptoms and Signs Approach to Differential Diagnosis and Treatment.* There are already a number of excellent textbooks in this field, but most focus on the diagnosis and work back toward the signs and symptoms. The goal of this book was to take the opposite approach—to start with presenting complaints and findings and guide the reader along the diagnostic pathway.

This book is intended for medical students, mid-level practitioners, residents, and fellows in neuromuscular medicine. I chose the authors of each chapter because they are all great clinician educators and writers, and I am extremely grateful for their contributions. I hope that by reading *Neuromuscular Disorders: A Symptoms and Signs Approach to Differential Diagnosis and Treatment,* you develop a greater enthusiasm and confidence in caring for your patients with neuromuscular disorders.

Nicholas J. Silvestri, MD

1 Interpretation of Tests Used in Neuromuscular Disorders

Diana Mnatsakanova and David Lacomis

The evaluation of patients with neuromuscular diseases usually requires a comprehensive approach that utilizes laboratory, electrodiagnostic, and sometimes histopathologic testing. However, the process starts with a detailed history and physical examination that guides localization, differential diagnosis, and test selection. The evaluator should keep in mind multiple potential levels of localization, including muscle, neuromuscular junction (NMJ), peripheral nerve, nerve root, and anterior horn of the spinal cord sites.

Hallmark but nonspecific clinical features include symmetric proximal weakness in myopathy with associated difficulty performing tasks such as combing hair, rising from a chair, and climbing stairs. Myalgias and muscle cramps can be present. In some myopathies, there are accompanying bulbar and ocular symptoms such as ptosis, dysphagia, and dysarthria. Patients with neuromuscular transmission disorders, such as myasthenia gravis (MG), may complain of fatigable weakness, ptosis, diplopia, dysarthria, dysphagia, and shortness of breath. Sensorimotor neuropathies usually present with sensory symptoms such as numbness and paresthesias, along with distal weakness and reflex loss. Hereditary neuropathies are not typically associated with pain and have a slowly progressive course. Patients with motor neuronopathies such as amyotrophic lateral sclerosis (ALS) present with asymmetric weakness, bulbar symptoms, and fasciculations. There is considerable overlap of many of these signs and symptoms among disorders of the motor unit.

Once the examiner has localized the lesion and formulated a working differential diagnosis, testing is pursued. In this chapter, we discuss the interpretation and utility of the most useful forms of testing in myopathy, neuropathy, NMJ disorders, and neuronopathies. Imaging is not covered.

LABORATORY TESTING
Serum Creatine Kinase
Neurologists are frequently consulted to evaluate elevated creatine kinase (CK) levels, regardless of whether there are accompanying symptoms of weakness.

- The MM isozyme of serum CK is predominantly produced by skeletal muscle, and serum CK levels reflect muscle membrane integrity.

CK is located in myofibrils and is also present in mitochondria. It plays a role in energy metabolism by catalyzing creatine and adenosine triphosphate (ATP) to phosphocreatine and adenosine diphosphate (ADP). CK levels become elevated if there is a muscle membrane leak or muscle necrosis.

- The normal range depends on the individual's muscle mass, race, sex, and activity levels.
- Vigorous exercise is associated with elevated CK levels, and it is important for the patient to stop exercising 5–7 days before CK levels are checked.

CK measurement is one of the most useful tests in neuromuscular disease, especially when myopathy is in the differential diagnosis. However, CK elevation is not specific to myopathy. Some neurogenic disorders, exercise, and trauma are among the conditions that elevate CK. A list of such processes is found in Table 1.1, along with the usual range of CK values. Additional descriptions of metabolic myopathies are found in the next subsection. Also, keep in mind that the CK level may be elevated in cardiac disease, but the MB fraction is most dramatically affected. Electrodiagnostic testing, muscle biopsy, and genetic testing may be considered for further evaluations following identification of an elevated CK (discussed later in the chapter).

- Aldolase, which is found in the liver as well as muscle, is elevated in most conditions in which the CK is elevated. An abnormally high level of aldolase may be seen in some inflammatory disorders affecting fascia in which the CK level is normal.

With regard to myopathy, other potentially useful laboratory testing is listed in Table 1.2.

Inherited Metabolic Myopathies
Metabolic myopathies are skeletal muscle disorders usually caused by abnormal metabolism of glucose and free fatty acids. Metabolic myopathies comprise glycogen-storage diseases, fatty acid oxidation defects, and mitochondrial myopathies. Clinical features suggestive of metabolic myopathies include myalgias associated with participation in endurance or power sports, rhabdomyolysis, myoglobinuria, symptoms triggered by fasting or systemic illness, or

TABLE 1.1 Causes of Elevated Creatine Kinase

Conditions	Frequency of CK elevation	Degree of CK elevation
Myopathies		
Inflammatory myopathies: PM, IBM, DM	Most	Moderate to high; less elevated in IBM
Necrotizing autoimmune myopathy	All	Very high
Some toxic myopathies (e.g., cholesterol-lowering agents, colchicine)	Common	Mild to high
Critical illness myopathy	At least 50%	Mild to high
Hypothyroid myopathy	Common	Mild to high
Muscular dystrophies	Common	Dystrophinopathies (very high); limb-girdle dystrophy (variable); myotonic dystrophy (normal to mild); facioscapulohumeral (normal to moderate); oculopharyngeal (normal to mild); distal (mild to very high)
Myofibrillar myopathy	Common	Normal to moderate
Some glycogen storage myopathies	Common	Mild to moderate[#]
Mitochondrial myopathy	Occasional	Mild to moderate
Carnitine deficiency; some other lipid myopathies	Occasional	Mild[#]
Congenital myopathy	Occasional	Mild
Rhabdomyolysis, including causes such as cocaine use	All	High to very high
Neurogenic disorders		
Motor neuron diseases	Occasional	Mild to moderate
	Common with X-linked SBMA	

(*continued*)

TABLE 1.1 Causes of Elevated Creatine Kinase (*continued*)

Conditions	Frequency of CK elevation	Degree of CK elevation
Other neurogenic disorders	Variable	Variable
Trauma (includes exercise, seizure)	Unknown	Variable
Neuroleptic malignant syndrome	Common	At least moderate
Malignant hyperthermia	Common	High or very high
MacroCPK (CK-IgG Ab)	About 1% general population	

Occasional = <25%; common = 25%–75%; most = >75%.
Mild = <4-fold; moderate = 4- to 10-fold; high = >10-fold; very high = >50-fold.
# Highly elevated during episodes of myoglobinuria.
Ab, antibody; DM, dermatomyositis; IBM, inclusion body myositis;
PM, polymyositis; SBMA, spinobulbar muscular atrophy.

TABLE 1.2 Other Laboratory Screening Tests for Myopathies and Their Significance

Laboratory screening test	Myopathies associated with test abnormality
Thyroid-stimulating hormone, other thyroid function tests	Hypothyroid myopathy Hyperthyroid myopathy
24-hour urinary free cortisol	Cushing syndrome
Serum protein electrophoresis	Amyloid myopathy; rod-body myopathy (monoclonal gammopathy) Inflammatory myopathy (hypergammaglobulinemia)
Myositis-associated antibodies: Anti-synthetases such as Jo-1 Signal recognition particle Mi-2 TIF-1 gamma	Anti-synthetase syndrome Necrotizing autoimmune myopathy Dermatomyositis Cancer-associated dermatomyositis
3-Hydroxy-3-methylglutaryl-CoA reductase (HMGCR) antibody	Necrotizing autoimmune myopathy
HIV antibody (Ab)	HIV
Alkaline phosphatase, calcium, phosphorus 25 OH-vitamin D, parathyroid hormone	Osteomalacia, hypovitaminosis D, parathyroid disorders (primary and secondary)

(*continued*)

TABLE 1.2 Other Laboratory Screening Tests for Myopathies and Their Significance (*continued*)

Laboratory screening test	Myopathies associated with test abnormality
Vitamin E	Vitamin E deficiency
Serum and urine carnitine levels	Carnitine deficiency (primary and secondary)
GAA (acid maltase) assay	Pompe disease
ESR, CRP, anti-nuclear Ab, Sjogren Abs, complement components C3, C4, PM-Scl Ab; U1 ribonucleoprotein Ab	Associated connective tissue diseases
Serum lactate, pyruvate	Mitochondrial myopathy
Acetyl carnitine assay by tandem mass spectrometry; urine organic acid	Fatty acid metabolism defects
Genetic testing: appropriate patients based on predictive clinical and EMG features and FH	Many

CRP, C-reactive protein; EMG, electromyography; ESR, erythrocyte sedimentation rate; FH, family history; HMGCr, 3-hydroxy-3-methylglutary-CoA.

nausea/vomiting associated with exercise. Common serum testing for metabolic myopathies include CK levels, serum acylcarnitine profile by tandem mass spectrometry, urine organic acids, uric acid, lactate, pyruvate, serum amino acids, and appropriate genetic testing.

1. *Glycogen storage diseases:* McArdle disease is the most common type of glycogen storage disease and is due to myophosphorylase deficiency. Other rare glycogen storage diseases include phosphofructokinase, lactate dehydrogenase, phosphorylase b kinase, phosphoglycerate mutase, aldolase A, β-enolase, phosphoglucomutase, and phosphoglycerate kinase 1 deficiencies. In contrast, Pompe disease (acid maltase or acid alpha-glucosidase [GAA] deficiency) is an intralysosomal glycogen storage disease that presents with proximal weakness and sometimes ventilatory failure in adults. In infants, it also causes cardiomyopathy. Diagnosis is made by identification of a low or absent GAA level in blood, autophagic vacuolar myopathy with glycogen storage histopathologically, and genetic testing for a *GAA* mutation. CK levels are always elevated in infantile Pompe disease, and they are usually elevated in the adult form.

2. *Diseases with fatty acid oxidation defects:* Carnitine palmitoyltransferase II deficiency, trifunctional protein deficiency, and very-long-chain acyl-CoA dehydrogenase deficiency are the three most common disorders associated with fatty acid oxidation defects.

3. *Mitochondrial myopathies:* This diverse group of disorders is characterized by a primary defect in electron transport chain function. Given mitochondria are present in most human tissues, clinical presentations of mitochondrial myopathies include multisystemic features. Some of the more common mitochondrial myopathies include mitochondrial encephalopathy, lactic acidosis, and stroke-like episodes (MELAS); myoclonic epilepsy with ragged red fibers (MERRF); chronic progressive external ophthalmoplegia (CPEO); Kearns-Sayre syndrome; complex IV deficiency; cytochrome b mutations; and cytochrome c oxidase mutations.

Other Laboratory Screening Tests for Myopathies

A summary of other useful testing for evaluating specific types of myopathies is found in Table 1.2.

Laboratory Testing in NMJ Disorders

Nerve depolarization allows calcium influx through the voltage-gated calcium channels (VGCCs), which results in release of acetylcholine into the synaptic cleft. Acetylcholine binds to its acetylcholine receptor (AChR), opening ACh/sodium channels, allowing for influx of sodium and depolarization of the muscle membrane.

1. *Myasthenia gravis:* The growing panel of antibody (Ab) assays has improved diagnosis of NMJ transmission disorders such as MG. There are three types of AChR Ab assays: binding, blocking, and modulating.
   - Binding AChR Abs are the most sensitive and specific and are present in 85% to 90% of patients with generalized MG.
   - Blocking AChR Abs are present in 50% of patients with generalized MG.
   - Modulating AChR Abs are present in about 85% of patients with generalized MG and increase the sensitivity of MG diagnosis by only 5%; that is, they are present in 5% of patients who are negative for AChR binding Ab.
   - AChR Abs are seen in 50% of patients with ocular MG.
   - AChR Abs correlate with thymic pathology (hyperplasia or a thymoma), but muscle-specific tyrosine kinase (MuSK) Abs do not (Table 1.3).
   - Of the 15% of patients with generalized MG who are negative for AChR Ab, 40% have MuSK Abs. MuSK Abs are usually not present in ocular MG.

   Patients with MuSK Abs can present with oculobulbar (diplopia, ptosis, and dysarthria) or "myopathic" forms (proximal weakness, neck extension weakness, and respiratory weakness) of MG. Antistriated muscle Abs are nonspecific and are present in about 36% of all patients with MG and in 80% of patients with thymoma

(Table 1.3). Some seronegative patients have Abs to LRP 4 (low-density lipoprotein receptor–related protein 4) or rapsyn, but commercial testing is not yet available for those two Abs.

2. ***Lambert-Eaton myasthenic syndrome (LEMS):*** This syndrome is much less common than MG, and it may be difficult to diagnose. Patients with LEMS present with proximal weakness, dysautonomia, hyporeflexia or areflexia, and infrequently respiratory involvement. In as many as 40% of patients, a previously absent deep tendon reflex will return to normal after 10 seconds of maximal voluntary contraction.

   • Clinical features of LEMS frequently precede a diagnosis of small cell lung cancer that is ultimately found in about two-thirds of patients.

TABLE 1.3 Laboratory Testing in Neuromuscular Junction Disorders

Antibody	Disorder	Frequency	Other
Acetylcholine receptor (binding type most useful)	Generalized MG	85%	Thymic hyperplasia <50 yo
	Ocular MG	50%	Thymus atrophy >50 yo
	LEMS	Rare	Thymoma 10%–15%
Muscle-specific kinase (MuSK)	Generalized MG	6%	Normal thymus
	Ocular MG	Rare?	
Seronegative (may have LRP4 or agrin Abs)*	Generalized MG	10%	No thymoma
	Ocular MG	48%	
Striated muscle (mainly titin Ab)	Late-onset MG	55%	With or without thymoma
	MG with thymoma (all ages)	54%	90% PPV in patients under 50 yo and 71% PPV in patients >50 yo
	Ocular MG	0.6%	Without thymoma
Voltage-gated calcium channel (P/Q > N>L types)	LEMS	85%–95%	With or without small cell lung cancer
	Paraneoplastic disorder without LEMS	44%	With cerebellar degeneration
	Small cell lung CA	28%	

*Testing is not yet commercially available.
CA, cancer; LEMS, Lambert-Eaton myasthenic syndrome; MG, myasthenia gravis; PPV, positive predictive value; yo, years old.

- VGCC antibodies are present in as many as 90% of patients with autoimmune LEMS and in 100% of patients with paraneoplastic LEMS.

3. **Botulism:** Botulism causes presynaptic NMJ dysfunction. It is largely a clinical diagnosis, and presenting symptoms include ocular and bulbar weakness, descending weakness, ventilatory dysfunction with prodromal syndrome of nausea, abdominal cramps, and diarrhea. Some patients develop autonomic dysfunction.

   - Diagnosis is confirmed by detection of serum, gastric, or stool toxin in addition to electrodiagnostic features of a presynaptic defect (discussed later), which may be subtle.

Laboratory Testing for Neuropathies

Neuropathy can be classified pathologically as neuronal (ganglion), axonal, demyelinating, or mixed axonal and demyelinating. It can also be classified by distribution: single nerve, multiple nerves, root, plexus, and polyneuropathy (PN). This is a vast topic. We will concentrate on axonal and demyelinating PN, but some conditions that cause PN may also affect a more restricted distribution of nerves. Some systemic causes are described here, and a summary of possible laboratory testing is provided in Table 1.4.

TABLE 1.4 Possible Laboratory Tests for Neuropathy

Laboratory screening test	Neuropathy associated with test abnormality
FBS, HbA1c, 2-hour OGTT*	Diabetic, prediabetic
TSH	Hypothyroid
Vitamin B_{12}*, methylmalonic acid*	Vitamin B_{12} deficiency
Folate	Folate deficiency
SPEP with immunofixation*; quantitative immunoglobulins; free light chains (serum)	Monoclonal gammopathies; POEMS (add vascular endothelial growth factor); primary amyloidosis
Human immunodeficiency virus (HIV) Ab	HIV
Vitamin E (low)	Vitamin E deficiency (sensory)
Vitamin B_6 (low or high)	Vitamin B_6 deficiency or toxicity (sensory)
ESR, CRP, ANA, RF, C3, C4, SS-A/B Abs; ANCA; cryoglobulins; hepatitis B and C screen	Associated connective tissue disease or systemic vasculitis
Myelin-associated glycoprotein (MAG) Ab; SGPG (sulfoglucuronyl paragloboside) Ab	Distal, symmetric, demyelinating sensory > motor PN

(continued)

TABLE 1.4 Possible Laboratory Tests for Neuropathy (*continued*)

Laboratory screening test	Neuropathy associated with test abnormality
Ganglioside GM1 IgM Ab	Multifocal motor neuropathy (50%+)
GQ1b Ab	Ataxic sensorimotor PN; ophthalmoplegia (Miller-Fisher syndrome)
Paraneoplastic Abs, especially anti-Hu (ANNA-1) and CV2	Sensory neuronopathy; sensory neuropathy
Copper (low)	Myeloneuropathy
Porphyrins: urine and stool	Porphyric: motor, sensory, dysautonomia; central nervous system
Heavy metals (e.g., lead, arsenic in urine and blood)	Heavy metal intoxication
Lyme titer (Western blot to confirm)	Lyme radiculopathy, mononeuropathy, polyneuropathy
Cerebrospinal fluid cells and protein	AIDP, CIDP (albuminocytologic disassociation); HIV, other viruses, sarcoid, neoplastic (cellular)
Genetic testing** (e.g., CMT1A: PMP22) Duplication/HNPP: PMP22 deletion; GJB1, MFN2	Charcot-Marie-Tooth disease Leukodystrophies with neuropathy Fabry disease

* Recommended by the American Academy of Neurology for screening distal symmetric PN.
** Recommended by the American Academy of Neurology for classifying hereditary neuropathies and some cryptogenic neuropathies with a hereditary neuropathy phenotype starting with the most common types or expected type based on clinical and electrodiagnostic features.
AIDP, acute inflammatory demyelinating PN; ANA, antinuclear Ab; ANCA, antineutrophilic cytoplasmic Ab; CIDP, chronic inflammatory demyelinating PN; CMT1A, Charcot-Marie-Tooth disease type IA; CRP, C-reactive protein; ESR, erythrocyte sedimentation rate; FBS, fasting blood sugar; GJB1, gap junction beta-1 protein; HbA1c, glycosylated hemoglobin; HNPP, hereditary neuropathy with liability to pressure palsies; MFN2, mitofusin 2; OGTT, oral glucose tolerance test; PN, polyneuropathy; RF, rheumatoid factor; TSH, thyroid-stimulating hormone.

Vitamin Deficiencies

Vitamin deficiencies often affect the peripheral nervous system (PNS), particularly nerves, in addition to other organs. The greater susceptibility of peripheral nerves to these deficiencies is likely due to the metabolic demands of long axons. Due to this phenomenon, clinical symptoms are typically associated with a symmetric and length-dependent axonal neuropathy. Clinical clues may include weight loss, malnutrition, alcoholism, symptoms of sprue, and history of gastric surgery that predispose to malabsorption.

- *Vitamin B_{12} deficiency* is typically characterized by signs of central and peripheral motor dysfunction, posterior column involvement, cognitive disturbances, and megaloblastic anemia in addition to axonal or mixed sensorimotor PN. A low serum B_{12} level confirms the diagnosis. Serum methylmalonic acid and homocysteine levels that are increased add about 5% to 10% sensitivity in patients whose B_{12} levels are normal.
- *Copper deficiency* presents similarly to vitamin B_{12} deficiency. Copper absorption is competitive with zinc absorption, and there have been reported cases showing association between zinc toxicity and copper deficiency.
- *Vitamin E deficiency* typically manifests as a spinocerebellar syndrome and large fiber sensory-predominant axonal PN.
- *Vitamin B_6 deficiency* typically occurs in the setting of isoniazid treatment for tuberculosis. Excess of vitamin B_6, which typically occurs with ingestion of megadoses of vitamin B_6 (>2 g/d), can lead to a sensory neuropathy as well.
- *Vitamin B_1 deficiency* typically presents with progressive axonal sensorimotor PN. Associated symptoms include cranial neuropathies and cognitive dysfunction. Measurement of B_1 blood levels may not be reliable. Erythrocyte transketolase assay may be more useful.

Systemic Disorders

The PNS is frequently affected by other systemic disorders. Such common disorders include diabetes mellitus (DM), endocrinopathies, and paraproteinemia. Neurosarcoidosis, systemic vasculitis, amyloidosis, neoplasia, and liver and kidney diseases may also affect the PNS, particularly the nerves, so they are mentioned here.

- *Diabetes mellitus:* DM is the most common cause of PN. Its effects on the nerves are widespread and include distal sensorimotor axonal or mixed PN (most common type), small fiber neuropathy, mononeuropathies, lumbosacral radiculoplexus neuropathy, thoracoabdominal radiculopathy, and autonomic neuropathy. Laboratory testing should include a fasting blood glucose and hemoglobin A1c levels. If negative, a 2-hour glucose tolerance test is useful, especially in detecting prediabetes. Peripheral neuropathy symptoms can precede a DM diagnosis.
- *Thyroid hormone disorders:* Both hypothyroidism and hyperthyroidism (thyrotoxicosis) can cause widespread neurologic problems ranging from cognitive dysfunction to nerve and muscle

involvement. Neuromuscular disorders associated with thyrotox-icosis include proximal myopathy, periodic paralysis, MG, and neuropathy. Hypothyroidism is typically associated with signs of muscle weakness, sensorimotor axonal neuropathy, and carpal tunnel syndrome. Serum workup for TSH, free T_4, and T_3 levels is suggested.

- *Adrenal hormone disorders:* Glucocorticoid excess (Cushing syndrome) is associated with neurologic complications such as proximal myopathy and cognitive dysfunction, while glucocorticoid deficiency (Addison disease) is typically associated with neuropsychiatric problems. Workup includes a 24-hour urine free cortisol level.

- *Neurosarcoidosis:* Neurosarcoidosis is associated with a broad range of clinical manifestations. Neuromuscular involvement is rare and mainly occurs via direct granulomatous infiltration or compression. Patients typically present with a painful non-length-dependent axonal PN or polyradiculoneuropathy. Other presentations include mononeuritis multiplex, entrapment syndromes, subacute demyelinating PN, small fiber neuropathy, dysautonomia, and peripheral nerve vasculitis. Serum angiotensin-converting enzyme (ACE) level is sometimes elevated, but due to its low sensitivity, diagnosis is made via tissue biopsy.

- *Systemic vasculitis:* A variety of chronic inflammatory conditions that include autoimmune attack on blood vessels cause peripheral nerve ischemic axonal degeneration. These disorders include rheumatoid arthritis, systemic lupus erythematosus, Sjögren syndrome, cryoglobulinemia, granulomatosis with polyangiitis (Wegener), eosinophilic granulomatosis with polyangiitis (Churg-Strauss), polyarteritis nodosa, and microscopic polyangiitis. The most common neuromuscular presentations of systemic vasculitis are overlapping mononeuropathies with PN and mononeuritis multiplex that manifest as painful, asymmetric, asynchronous sensorimotor axonal neuropathy. Serum workup is outlined in Table 1.4.

- *Paraproteinemia:* Monoclonal gammopathies are common in patients with PN. M proteins are produced by B lymphocytes or plasma cells and are composed of a heavy chain (immunoglobulin IgG, IgA, IgM, IgD, or IgE) and a light chain (kappa and lambda). Neuropathies associated with paraproteinemias include distal acquired demyelinating sensory (DADS) with M protein (a chronic inflammatory demyelinating polyneuropathy [CIDP] variant); Waldenström macroglobulinemia; multiple myeloma; PN, organomegaly, endocrinopathy, monoclonal plasma cell disorder, and skin changes (POEMS) syndrome; primary systemic amyloidosis; and monoclonal gammopathy of undetermined significance (MGUS). Laboratory evaluation for monoclonal gammopathy includes serum protein electrophoresis (SPEP) with serum immunofixation (Table 1.4). Approximately 50% of patients with DADS have antibodies to myelin-associated glycoprotein (MAG).

- *Paraneoplastic neuropathies:* These rare neuroimmunologic disorders occur in a minority of patients with cancer. Paraneoplastic neuropathies include sensory neuronopathy (sensory ganglionopathy), autonomic neuropathy, demyelinating neuropathy, and rarely motor neuropathy. Sensory ganglionopathy commonly presents with upper limb sensory ataxia and is associated with dysautonomia and usually antineuronal nuclear Ab type 1 (ANNA-1 or Hu). It most commonly occurs with small cell lung cancer. Other paraneoplastic antibodies include anti-CV2 (collapsin response mediator protein-5 [CRMP-5]), anti-Yo (Purkinje cell antibody-1 [PCA-1]), anti-Ri (ANNA-2), anti-amphiphysin, anti-ganglionic nicotinic AChR, anti-voltage-gated potassium channel complex, and anti-VGCC (N type) antibodies.

Infectious Etiologies

PNS infections have broad manifestations, including ganglionopathy, cranial neuropathies, polyradiculopathy, mononeuritis multiplex, and PN.

- *Herpes viruses:* Herpes simplex virus 1 and 2 (HSV1, HSV2) and varicella zoster virus (VZV) account for some PNS infections. Following the primary infection of chickenpox, VZV remains dormant in the dorsal root ganglia. Subsequent reactivation of VZV results in herpes zoster (shingles), which presents as a painful vesicular rash in the dermatomal sensory distribution. Postherpetic neuralgia is a neuropathic pain in the distribution of previous rash.
- *Human immunodeficiency virus (HIV):* HIV typically presents with symmetric length-dependent axonal sensorimotor PN and sometimes sensory neuropathy. Acute inflammatory polyradiculoneuropathy (AIDP) can occur around the time of seroconversion.
- *Hepatitis C:* Multiple types of PN are attributed to hepatitis C virus, including length-dependent sensorimotor axonal PN, mononeuritis multiplex, and rarely demyelinating inflammatory neuropathy. Mixed cryoglobulinemia is commonly associated with hepatitis C virus.
- *West Nile virus (WNV):* In addition to encephalitis, WNV can present as motor paralysis due to anterior horn cell involvement. Motor neuropathy can begin asymmetrically but typically generalizes. Respiratory involvement is common and may require invasive ventilation.
- *Lyme disease:* This infectious disease is caused by the *Borrelia burgdorferi* spirochete. Early neurologic symptoms include meningitis, cranial neuritis, radiculoneuritis, and cardiac manifestations. Late-stage neurologic manifestations include axonal

polyradiculoneuropathy and encephalomyelitis. Serologic testing includes IgM/IgG titers from ELISA; positive results are confirmed with a Western blot.

Acquired Immune Neuropathies

The members of this group of overlapping disorders share common motor, sensory, autoimmune, laboratory, and electrodiagnostic features. It is important to recognize them, as they are generally responsive to immunosuppressive therapies. Diagnosis is typically based on the clinical history, exam, electrodiagnostic studies, and presence of albuminocytologic dissociation in the cerebrospinal fluid (CSF). Antibodies, particularly against gangliosides, associated with this group of disorders typically have low sensitivity for diagnosis; however, they may be somewhat useful at least in the Miller-Fisher variant of Guillain-Barré syndrome (GBS).

- *Guillain-Barré syndrome:* GBS is an acute, monophasic, immune-mediated polyradiculoneuropathy with symptom nadir by 4 weeks from symptom onset. Acute inflammatory demyelinating polyradiculoneuropathy is the most common variant of GBS. Other forms include bifacial weakness with distal paresthesia, pharyngeal–cervical–brachial weakness, paraparetic variant with pain, Miller Fisher syndrome (associated with GQ1b antibodies), acute motor axonal neuropathy (associated with GM1 antibodies), acute motor sensory axonal neuropathy, and acute pandysautonomia. The CSF contains few or no cells with an elevated protein level (albuminocytologic disassociation).

- *Chronic-acquired demyelinating polyneuropathies:* These immune-mediated neuropathies share common features and are chronic in nature. Subcategories include CIDP, DADS neuropathy, and multifocal acquired demyelinating sensory and motor neuropathy (MADSAM). Multifocal motor neuropathy (MMN) may be a variant or close relative. Similar to GBS, the diagnosis of CIDP is suggested by CSF albuminocytologic dissociation in addition to history, exam, and electrodiagnostic findings and a course of progression beyond 8 weeks. MMN is a demyelinating motor neuropathy that typically presents with asymmetric limb weakness and manifests as a conduction block on electrodiagnostic testing. Approximately 50% of patients with MMN have elevated anti-GM1 antibodies. Patients with DADS have a distal symmetric phenotype and are typically associated with an elevated monoclonal protein level, but some do not have paraproteinemia.

Inherited Neuropathies

There are numerous forms of inherited neuropathy, most of which are classified as Charcot-Marie-Tooth disease type 1 (dysmyelinating) or type 2 (axonal), or as X-linked and intermediate forms that are well beyond the scope of this chapter. Diagnosis is based on clinical, exam, electrodiagnostic testing, and genetic testing (see the genetic testing section later in this chapter). *Transthyretin (TTR) familial amyloid PN* is due to *TTR* gene mutations and manifests as neuropathy, cardiomyopathy, and sometimes ocular disease. Patients typically present with small fiber neuropathy evolving to large fiber sensorimotor neuropathy and dysautonomia. They may have cardiomyopathy, gastrointestinal, and genitourinary involvement. *TTR* gene testing confirms the diagnosis; tissue biopsies of various organs can reveal amyloid deposition.

GENETIC TESTING

Introduction

In many inherited neuromuscular diseases, especially muscular dystrophies, genetic testing is usually required to confirm or make the diagnosis, especially in disorders with overlap in phenotypes from mutations in different genes (e.g., limb-girdle dystrophy) or with phenotypic variability from mutations involving the same gene (e.g., dysferlinopathy). In some instances, a specific type of mutation may be amenable to treatment—for example, exon skipping in Duchenne muscular dystrophy. Genetic testing is also useful for other inherited myopathies, inherited polyneuropathies, genetic forms of ALS, and congenital myasthenia.

This topic is vast and complex regarding the types of testing and mutations. There are also financial issues regarding insurance coverage for genetic testing, and ethical issues including those regarding testing of asymptomatic individuals at risk. The types of testing include testing of a single gene by polymerase chain reaction (PCR) or another analysis, testing of a targeted gene panel by various techniques including PCR and Sanger sequencing, next-generation sequencing comprehensive gene panels, comparative genomic hybridization arrays for analysis of duplications and deletions, and exome sequencing. Reviewing the techniques and their interpretation is beyond the scope of this chapter, and interpretation may involve consulting with the geneticist at the testing laboratory. Examples of some of the more common adult-onset disorders are provided here.

- *Myotonic dystrophies:* When examination findings reveal clinical myotonia (difficulty with muscle relaxation), weakness (proximal, distal, or bulbar), early cataracts, and cardiac abnormalities with strong family history of cataracts or muscle disease, one must suspect myotonic dystrophy (type 1 or 2). Myotonic dystrophy type 1 is autosomal dominant (AD) and due to expansions of CTG trinucleotide repeats on the *DMPK* gene. Myotonic dystrophy type 2 is due to expansions of CCTG tetranucleotide repeats on the *CNBP* gene. It is usually milder than type 1, involves proximal rather than distal muscles, and is often accompanied by pain.

- *Fascioscapulohumeral muscular dystrophy (FSHD):* This AD condition presents with slowly progressive asymmetric weakness of facial, periscapular, tibialis anterior, quadriceps, and abdominal muscles. It is associated with contraction of the macrosatellite repeat array D4Z4 in the subtelomere of chromosome 4q.
- *Channelopathies with myotonia:* These nondystrophic myotonias are caused by mutations in voltage-gated ion channels on the skeletal muscle membrane, resulting in myotonia and episodes of weakness. Sodium channelopathies—hyperkalemic periodic paralysis and paramyotonia congenita—have *SCN4A* gene mutations, whereas chloride channelopathies (myotonia congenita) are associated with *CLCN1* mutations.
- *Limb-girdle muscular dystrophies (LGMDs):* This heterogeneous group of genetic disorders is characterized by weakness of the shoulder and pelvic girdle muscles. If LGMD is suspected, one can order a LGMD panel to evaluate multiple genes.
- *Hereditary neuropathies:* It is important to suspect hereditary sensorimotor neuropathies when evaluating patients with distal symmetric neuropathies, especially with pes cavus. These typically present in childhood or teenage years but may be diagnosed much later. Many are AD. Patients may complain of distal weakness, numbness, foot-drop, hand weakness, and poor balance. The majority of genetic polyneuropathies are variants of Charcot-Marie-Tooth (CMT) disease. Family history and electrodiagnostic studies help differentiate between the various types of CMT. The most common form of CMT is the demyelinating form associated with peripheral myelin protein 22 (PMP22) gene duplication (CMT1A). The most common axonal form of CMT is CMT2A, which is associated with a mitochondrial fusion protein defect from a mitofusin 2 *(MFN2)* gene mutation. X-linked CMT is typically associated with the gap junction protein beta 1 *(GJB1)* gene. PMP22 gene deletion is associated with hereditary neuropathy with liability to pressure palsies (HNPP), in which patients complain of nerve entrapment syndromes.

Utility of Genetic Testing

When the clinical presentation lacks features suggesting a single disorder or a group of disorders—as occurs, for example, with myotonic disorders—a comprehensive genetic approach is more likely to be successful. With inherited neuropathies, the clinical and electrophysiologic features can be utilized to streamline the genetic testing.

When a known pathogenic mutation is identified, the test is "diagnostic." If a known benign polymorphism is identified, then the test would be considered negative. However, if the testing identifies a variant that has not been previously identified or is not known to be pathologic, it is usually reported as a variant of unknown significance. Testing of affected and unaffected family members, if feasible, or later association of the variant with the disease state in others may help determine whether the variant is clinically significant. If a test is negative, it must be known if it was a comprehensive test for the diseases/mutations in question. For example, were the methods adequate to detect a trinucleotide repeat or mutation in a noncoding region?

ELECTRODIAGNOSTIC TESTING

Introduction

In addition to the history, neurologic examination, and laboratory studies, electrodiagnostic testing (EDx) facilitates localization of neuromuscular disease. EDx is particularly useful in disorders that involve the motor unit. Recall that the motor unit consists of an anterior horn cell, its motor axons, NMJs, and innervated muscle fibers. Uncovering various electrodiagnostic patterns of neuropathic and myopathic processes as well as NMJ disorders can lead to more targeted laboratory testing and a refined differential diagnosis. These patterns are summarized in Table 1.5 and discussed in this section.

EDx testing may also be used to detect subclinical disorders, assess disease activity, and help select a suitable muscle or nerve for biopsy. EDx testing is guided by the history and neurologic examination findings.

Nerve Conduction Studies (NCS): Sensory Nerves

- Sensory nerve conduction studies evaluate the pathway from the dorsal root ganglion to the sensory receptor.
- A pure sensory nerve or mixed sensory and motor nerve is stimulated and depolarized, and the sensory nerve action potential (SNAP) is recorded from a pure sensory or sometimes a mixed nerve.
- Usually, recording electrodes are placed over a pure sensory nerve, and antidromic stimulation (against the usual direction of travel) is performed, since it is technically preferable.

Sensory responses are affected only by disturbances in larger nerve fibers at or distal to the dorsal root ganglion. Since radiculopathies are more proximal and typically do not involve the dorsal root ganglia, sensory responses are normal even in the presence of significant sensory loss clinically. Sensory responses are also normal with spinal cord sensory pathway involvement.

- Processes that affect sensory neurons or their *axons* will result in a reduction of the SNAP amplitude.
- The pattern of axonal involvement is then determined—namely, whether it is affecting a single nerve, multiple nerves, or the brachial or lumbosacral plexus.
- A length-dependent pattern is typical of most axonal polyneuropathies, but a non-length-dependent pattern may be seen in some ischemic disorders such as vasculitis or diabetes.

TABLE 1.5 Typical Electrodiagnostic Findings in Disorders of the Motor Unit

Disorder	SNAPs	CMAPs	Other	PSW/fibs	Small MUPs	Large MUPs	MUP recruit	Other
Myopathy	N	N or dec amp		+ or −	+	−	Incr	Myotonia, CRDs in some
Presynaptic NMJ	N	Dec amp	Incr RNS	−*	+ or −	−	N, dec	
Postsynaptic NMJ	N	N or dec amp	Decr RNS	−*	+ or −	−	N, dec	
Plexus	Dec amp	Dec amp		+	−	+	Dec	
Radiculopathy	N	N or dec amp		+	−	+	Dec	Myotomal pattern
Axonal SM PN	Dec amp	Dec amp	Mildly slow	+	−	+	Dec	
Demyelinating SM PN	Dec amp; inc DL	Dec amp; CB; temp disp	Inc DL; slow; long F-waves	−**	−‡	+**	Dec	
Small fiber PN	N	N		−	−	−	N	
Motor neuron disease	N	Dec amp		+	−‡	+	Dec	Fasciculation potentials

* Occasionally present, ** present with concomitant axonal degeneration, ‡ present with early reinnervation, + is present, − is absent. CB, conduction block; CMAPs, compound muscle action potentials; CRD, complex repetitive discharge; decr, decreased; decr, decrement with slow repetitive stimulation; disp, temporal dispersion; DL, distal latency; Fibs, fibrillation potentials; incr, increment with 10-s exercise or rapid repetitive stimulation; MUP, motor unit potential; N, normal; NMJ, neuromuscular junction; PN, peripheral neuropathy; PSW, positive sharp wave; RNS, repetitive nerve stimulation; SM, sensorimotor; SNAPs, sensory nerve action potentials.

- Pure sensory neuropathies are associated with paraneoplastic syndromes, Sjögren syndrome, a postinfectious process, some toxins, and vitamin B_6 intoxication.
- Disorders that cause demyelination or remyelination lead to prolongation of latencies and significant slowing of conduction velocities.
- Since the onset latency and conduction velocity depend primarily on the presence and function of the largest myelinated fibers, axonal neuropathies do not result in a significant reduction of conduction velocity until there has been marked loss of such fibers.
- In demyelinating disorders, there is loss of amplitude if the axons are not depolarized due to conduction block.
- Patients with pure small fiber PN have completely normal electrophysiologic studies.

Nerve Conduction Studies (NCS): Motor Nerves

Motor nerve cell bodies are located in the anterior horn of the spinal cord, extending peripherally toward the NMJ and muscle. Motor conduction studies are performed by stimulation of a mixed or sometimes pure motor nerve while recording over the innervated muscle as a compound muscle action potential (CMAP). Therefore, a motor response can be affected not only by a neuropathic process, but also by dysfunction of NMJs and muscle. The pathway that is examined begins at the anterior horn cell and ends at the muscle.

- The patterns seen with motor axonal loss (low amplitudes and mild or no slowing of conduction velocity) and demyelination (prolonged latencies, more severe slowing of conduction velocity, and possibly low amplitudes) are similar to those mentioned for sensory studies, except that the additional features described next may be present in CMAP morphology in demyelinating disorders.
- Conduction block, for example, is not reliably detected with sensory responses, which normally exhibit a proximal drop in amplitude while stimulating the same nerve mostly due to phase cancellation of the positive and negative components of the SNAP. This phenomenon is not substantially present in motor nerves. Therefore, if there is a block in conduction, usually due to demyelination, a drop in amplitude proximal to the affected region may be identified in the motor studies.
- In addition, there may be temporal dispersion due to differential slowing of individual nerve action potentials that summate to form the CMAP, especially with disorders associated with remyelination (Figure 1.1).
- Nerve conduction studies can be also used to distinguish between acquired and inherited demyelinating neuropathies. In inherited conditions, all myelin is affected equally, making conduction

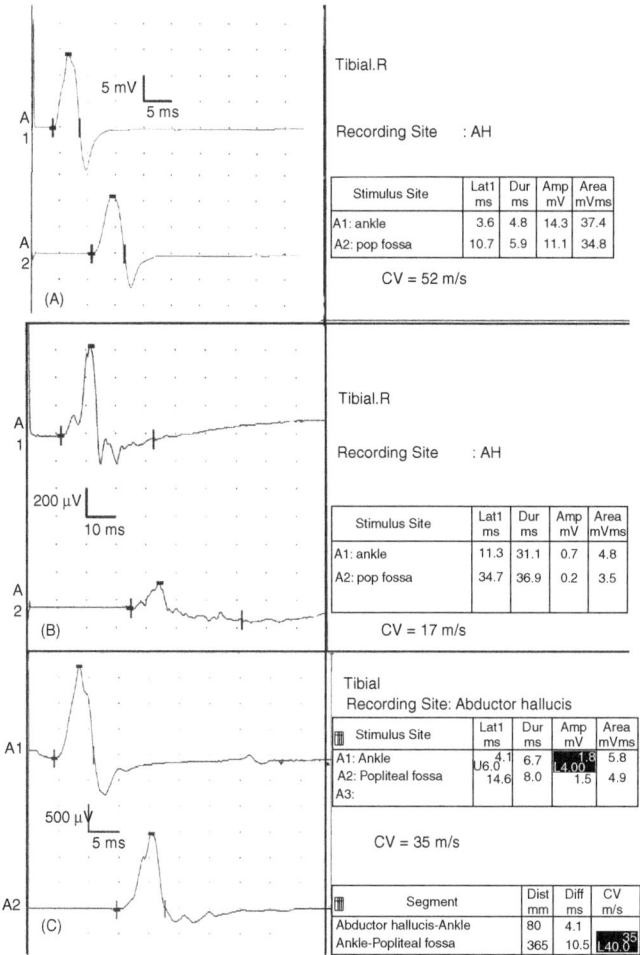

Panel (A) — Tibial.R

Recording Site : AH

Stimulus Site	Lat1 ms	Dur ms	Amp mV	Area mVms
A1: ankle	3.6	4.8	14.3	37.4
A2: pop fossa	10.7	5.9	11.1	34.8

CV = 52 m/s

Panel (B) — Tibial.R

Recording Site : AH

Stimulus Site	Lat1 ms	Dur ms	Amp mV	Area mVms
A1: ankle	11.3	31.1	0.7	4.8
A2: pop fossa	34.7	36.9	0.2	3.5

CV = 17 m/s

Panel (C) — Tibial

Recording Site: Abductor hallucis

Stimulus Site	Lat1 ms	Dur ms	Amp mV	Area mVms
A1: Ankle	6.0, 4.1	6.7	4.00, 1.8	5.8
A2: Popliteal fossa	14.6	8.0	1.5	4.9
A3:				

CV = 35 m/s

Segment	Dist mm	Diff ms	CV m/s
Abductor hallucis-Ankle	80	4.1	
Ankle-Popliteal fossa	365	10.5	40.0, 35

FIGURE 1.1 (A) Normal tibial motor NCS stimulating at the ankle (A1) and popliteal fossa (A2) and recording at the abductor hallucis. In most motor nerves, the proximal amplitude should not drop more than 20% compared to the distal CMAP, but a 50% drop is considered normal in the tibial nerve. (B) Tibial NCS from a patient with chronic inflammatory demyelinating PN. The distal latency with the takeoff marked in A1 is prolonged at 11.3 ms, with normal being less than 6.0 ms. The distal amplitude is low and the waveform is dispersed. With stimulation proximally at the popliteal fossa (A2), there is a significant drop in amplitude with temporal dispersion of the waveform due to demyelination. The conduction velocity is markedly slow at 17 m/s, with normal being greater than 40 m/s. (C) Tibial NCS from a patient with an axonal PN due to chemotherapy. The amplitudes are low as recorded from both stimulation sites without a significant proximal drop in amplitude. There is no significant temporal dispersion. The latency is normal and the conduction velocity is only mildly slow (35 m/s).

CMAP, compound muscle action potential; NCS, nerve conduction studies; PN, polyneuropathy.

velocities uniformly slow, and most do not exhibit temporal dispersion. In acquired conditions (GBS), demyelination is not uniform and may be asymmetric, resulting in conduction block and temporal dispersion.

- Acute polyneuropathies are infrequent, with the most common type being GBS. NCS may be normal in the first week even if there is axonal degeneration.

The findings of the sensory and motor NCS are then combined to determine whether there is dysfunction of a single nerve or multiple nerves, or if there is a sensorimotor disturbance or pure motor or pure sensory disturbances. With polyneuropathies, the patterns of symmetric length dependent, asymmetric length dependent, and non-length dependent should be sought. Lack of symmetry usually excludes a large number of toxic, metabolic, and genetic conditions.

Multiple single-nerve involvement occurs in mononeuritis multiplex most often due to vasculitis. Vasculitis may also cause asymmetric length-dependent or non-length-dependent axonal neuropathy patterns. Multiple pure motor nerve involvement occurs in MMN. In general, if there is a pure motor disturbance, then one must determine if it is more likely due to a neuropathic process, an anterior horn cell, or a NMJ or muscle disorder. If the disorder causes conduction block, temporal dispersion, or significant slowing of the conduction velocity, it is due to a demyelinating neuropathy. However, if it manifests as only a loss of amplitude, there are multiple possible explanations.

- In the setting of low motor and normal sensory responses, patients will need to be further evaluated for a NMJ disorder, especially LEMS.
- The most useful diagnostic test is the LEMS test, which is a CMAP elicited from a single, supramaximal stimulation administered before and after 10 seconds of exercise. In patients with LEMS, there tends to be a significant increment of greater than 100%. Even smaller increments should raise suspicion and lead to more extensive evaluation of motor nerves.
- Slower repetitive nerve stimulation (RNS) at 2 to 3 Hz may also be performed to screen for disorders of the NMJs.
- Both postsynaptic and presynaptic disorders can cause an abnormal (usually more than 10%) decremental response at slow rates.
- The yield, especially for MG, increases to about 85% with stimulation of proximal nerves such as spinal accessory and facial motor nerves, but RNS of distal nerves, such as the ulnar, is technically easier.
- With presynaptic disorders, rapid RNS (more than 20 Hz) may also be performed, especially when the standard LEMS test is not feasible, to assess for an incremental response.

**Needle Electrode Examination: Insertional and
Spontaneous Activity**

The next step component of EDx testing is the needle examination.
Needle EMG helps ascertain the chronicity of the disease and dif-
ferentiates between neurogenic versus myopathic underlying processes. Four components are evaluated:

- Insertional activity
- Spontaneous activity
- Motor unit potential (MUP) morphology
- MUP recruitment

Insertional activity is due to mechanical irritation of muscle fibers
by the needle electrode, resulting in a brief burst of electrical activity.

- If muscle has been replaced by adipose tissue or if muscle is not
  depolarizing, such as during an attack of periodic paralysis, insertional activity is decreased or absent.
- If there is irritation of either the motor end-plate or the postsynaptic membrane region, insertional activity is increased, usually
  in the form of positive sharp waves. Myotonic discharges may
  follow in a minority of cases (as discussed later in this section).

Different forms of abnormal *spontaneous activity* may occur
following a pause in needle movement. Positive sharp waves and
fibrillation potentials (Figure 1.2) occur in myopathic disorders in

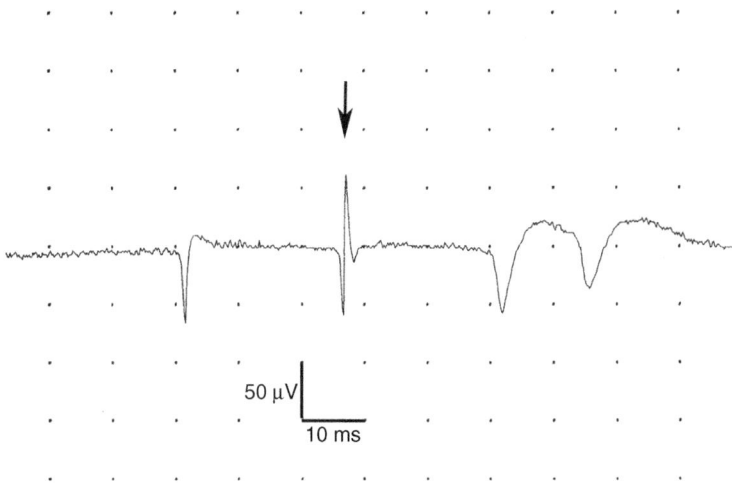

FIGURE 1.2 These positive sharp waves and a fibrillation potential (arrow) were
recorded from a denervated muscle at rest.

which there is muscle inflammation, muscle membrane dysfunction, or partial necrosis of myofibers. They also occur in neuropathic disorders in which there is denervation at the motor end-plate from any cause. They sometimes occur in more severe forms of NMJ dysfunction, especially botulism. Muscle trauma is another unusual cause.

- Spontaneous activity may be contiguous with increased insertional activity and includes positive sharp waves and fibrillation potentials. They fire regularly.
- Fasciculation potentials are another form of spontaneous activity. They have the appearance of a MUP (discussed later) but occur at rest and fire randomly. They are due to spontaneous depolarization of muscle fibers within a motor unit. The generator of fasciculation potentials can occur anywhere along the lower motor neuron pathways, from the anterior horn cell to the motor nerve terminal. When they are widespread, these potentials are more likely to be due to a disorder of anterior horn cells, but they are nonspecific (Figure 1.3).
- Myokymic discharges also appear spontaneously as groups of rhythmically firing MUPs that tend to sound like marching soldiers. The number of potentials within the group is highly variable and the firing pattern is semi-rhythmic. Myokymic discharges arise predominately in motor axons. They are nonspecific but may be seen in various neuropathic processes. They are characteristic of radiation-induced nerve injury.

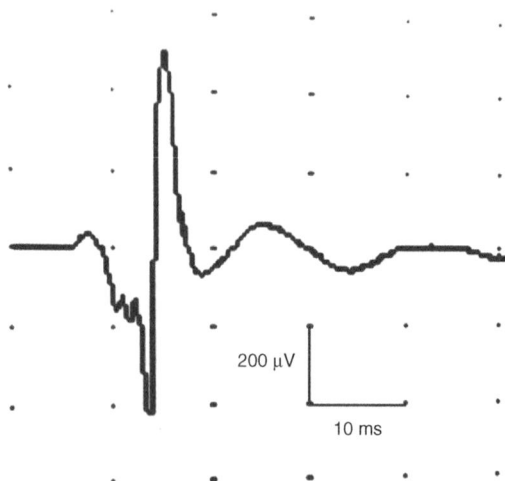

200 µV

10 ms

FIGURE 1.3 This fasciculation potential was recorded from a muscle (at rest) in a patient with amyotrophic lateral sclerosis.

- Other abnormal spontaneous activities include myotonic discharges, complex repetitive discharges (CRDs), and neuromyotonia.

Myotonic discharges:

- Consist of spikes or positive waves that wax and wane in amplitude and frequency or sometimes simply wane.
- Sound like a motorcycle engine revving—accelerating and decelerating.
- Emanate from the muscle membrane of single myofibers and are associated with myotonic dystrophies, myotonia congenita, and other channelopathies. In the myotonic dystrophies, there are also small motor potentials.

If myotonic discharges are prominent, consider one of the disorders shown in Table 1.6. Some are associated with the "myopathic" (short duration, low amplitude) MUPs described later in this chapter, while others are not.

Complex repetitive discharges (CRDs):

- Begin and end abruptly. There may be some change in morphology and amplitude during the recording, but the discharge has a period in which it is fires regularly.
- Have complexity that manifests as multiple phases or turns because of ephaptic transmission within groups of muscle fibers.

TABLE 1.6 Disorders With Prominent Myotonic Discharges

With "Myopathic" MUPs	Comment
Myotonic dystrophy type 1	Discharges typically wax and wane
Myotonic dystrophy type 2	Discharges commonly wane; sometimes only in paraspinals
Acid maltase (Pompe)/debrancher deficiency	Usually with CRDs
Toxic myopathy	
Cholesterol-lowering agents	Usually more focal
Hydroxychloroquine	May have axonal neuropathy
Colchicine	Often with axonal sensorimotor neuropathy
Without "Myopathic" MUPs	**Comment**
Myotonia congenita	Widespread with sodium-channel mutations
Hyperkalemic periodic paralysis	
Paramyotonia congenital	Widespread, profuse myotonia; worse with cooling
CRD, complex repetitive discharge; MUP, motor unit potential.	

- Sound more like a motor boat engine and are machinery like.
- Tend to be associated with conditions linked to muscle fiber split-ting, including some chronic myopathic and neurogenic disorders.
- Myopathies that may have prominent CRDs include acid maltase (Pompe), debrancher deficiencies, myofibrillar myopathy, and centronuclear myopathy.

Neuromyotonia is rare and consists of very rapidly firing (100–300 Hz) discharges that are continuous or occur in waves, sometimes with declining amplitudes. These discharges are due to peripheral nerve hyperexcitability states such as Isaac syndrome.

Needle Electrode Examination: MUP Morphology
MUPs are the summation of individual muscle fiber action potentials from myofibers within a motor unit.

- The main MUP features that are evaluated are duration, amplitude, and phases (baseline crossing plus one; Figure 1.4).

Normal durations vary somewhat among normal muscle groups, with facial muscles tending to have the shortest durations and muscles with a larger number of myofibers per motor unit, such as the gastrocnemius, tending to have longer-duration MUPs. MUP duration and amplitude also increase with age.

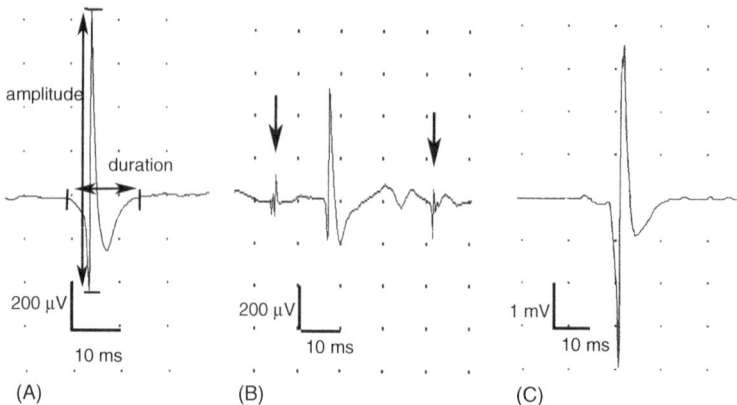

FIGURE 1.4 (A) A normal motor unit potential (MUP) is shown. The duration is the region from baseline crossing to baseline crossing; the amplitude is measured from the downward positive peak to the upward negative peak. (B) Two low-amplitude, short-duration, polyphasic MUPs are seen from a patient with inclusion body myositis. (C) A very-high-amplitude, long-duration MUP is shown from a patient with a history of polio. Note that the gain is 1 mv per division, while the gain in A and B is only 200 mv per division. All recordings are from the vastus lateralis.

- In myopathic processes, MUPs become shorter in duration and often have a low amplitude because of loss, atrophy, or dysfunction of muscle fibers within the motor unit (Figure 1.4).
- MUPs may become polyphasic due to loss of synchrony of depolarization of muscle fibers within the motor unit, especially in the more chronic myopathic conditions.
- The differential diagnosis for an EMG finding of small MUPs with fibrillation potentials differs from that of small MUPs without fibrillation potentials, but there is overlap (Tables 1.7 and 1.8).
- Small MUPs with fibrillation potentials may also occur with botulism and potentially with muscle trauma.
- In neurogenic processes, MUPs become enlarged—they have high amplitude and long duration—during the process of reinnervation, as sprouting axons bring more muscle fibers into the motor unit (Figure 1.4).
- With early reinnervation, there is a transition period in which MUPs may be small, electrically unstable, and polyphasic due to immature axon sprouts with unstable NMJs.
- In PN, there is a characteristic distal to proximal gradient of neuropathic MUP changes, where distal muscles are more affected than the proximal muscles. In radiculopathy, the findings follow a myotomal pattern

TABLE 1.7 "Myopathic" MUPs With Fibrillation Potentials

Category of myopathies	Examples
Inflammatory	Polymyositis Dermatomyositis Inclusion body myositis Necrotizing autoimmune myopathy Sarcoid myopathy/granulomatous myositis
Toxic	Cholesterol-lowering agents
ICU acquired	Critical illness myopathy
Endocrine	Hypothyroid myopathy
Dystrophies	Dystrophinopathies (occasional) Some limb-girdle muscular dystrophies Myofibrillar myopathies (some also have prominent CRDs) Distal dystrophies (common with desminopathy) FSHD (uncommon)
Infiltrative	Amyloid myopathy
Congenital	Centronuclear and myotubular (occasionally)
Metabolic	Carnitine deficiency Acid maltase and debrancher deficiencies Mitochondrial (some)

CRD, complex repetitive discharge; FSHD, facioscapulohumeral muscular dystrophy; MUP, motor unit potential.

TABLE 1.8 Myopathic MUPs Without Fibrillation Potentials

Category of myopathies	Examples
Treated inflammatory/autoimmune	Polymyositis Dermatomyositis
Infiltrative	Amyloid myopathy
Toxic	Corticosteroid myopathy
ICU acquired	Critical Illness myopathy (about half)
Endocrine	Cushing syndrome Hyperthyroidism Hypothyroidism (some)
Dystrophies	LGMD (e.g., LGMD2A and LGMD2B) Oculopharyngeal muscular dystrophy FSHD Bethlem myopathy Distal (some) Myofibrillar myopathy (some)
Congenital	Congenital myopathy (most)
Metabolic	Mitochondrial myopathy (some) Glycogen storage diseases (lysosomal types, some; non-lysosomal types, most) Lipid storage diseases Carnitine deficiency (some) Carnitine palmityl transferase (CPT) deficiency (most)

FSHD, fascioscapulohumeral muscular dystrophy; LGMD, limb-girdle muscular dystrophies; MUP, motor unit potential.

- In chronic myopathies, such as inclusion body myositis, there may also be enlarged MUPs.
- In some myopathies, EMG may be normal, including some cases of corticosteroid, mitochondrial, congenital, and inherited metabolic myopathies.
- In most myopathies, abnormal MUPs are often more prominent in proximal and paraspinal muscles, but the findings may be patchy.

Needle Electrode Examination: Recruitment

Recruitment refers to the firing rate for a given number of MUPs being activated at a certain degree of force; smaller MUPs become activated before larger MUPs. When a single MUP is activated and muscle contraction increases, the firing rate will increase up to 8–10 Hz, and then a second MUP will be recruited.

- In myopathic processes, a larger number of MUPs is recruited to generate the same degree of force as in a normal muscle.
- Therefore, in myopathic processes, recruitment is early (also called rapid or increased). The firing rate of the MUPs is within the normal range.

- In contrast, in neurogenic processes, recruitment is decreased since there is loss of MUPs; the remaining MUPs must fire at an increased rate (more than 15Hz) to compensate for this loss. Recruitment may also be decreased in an end-stage myopathic process due to few myofibers remaining in the motor unit.
- Patients with pain may not activate a muscle such that few MUPs fire, but the firing rate is normal. This phenomenon of *decreased activation* must be distinguished from decreased recruitment in which the firing rate increases.
- Decreased activation also occurs in upper motor neuron processes.

MUSCLE AND NERVE BIOPSY

Muscle Biopsy

Introduction

Biopsy of skeletal muscle is an important component of the evaluation of many patients with myopathy. When interpreting the biopsy report, including the microscopic description, it is important to first make a judgment as to whether the correct muscle was selected for biopsy, and whether it is representative of the patient's disorder. If the biopsy site was not well chosen, the findings may not be clinically relevant. It is also important that the pathologist had access to the history so that the proper evaluation was performed. Finally, it should be noted whether the interpretation was compromised by factors such as significant artifact.

Major Histopathologic Diagnoses

The following major histopathologic diagnoses are typically made:

1. Myopathy/myopathic change
2. Neurogenic atrophy
3. Type II fiber atrophy
4. No specific or diagnostic histopathologic findings

There are subgroups and variations for all of these diagnoses. Most histopathologic findings are actually nonspecific.

Myopathic Histopathologic Findings

In general, myopathic changes may begin with *myofiber degeneration or necrosis* in which the myofiber cytoplasm (sarcoplasm) becomes pale and disintegrates. Macrophages then infiltrate the sarcoplasm in the process of *myophagocytosis* (Figure 1.5).

Regenerating myofibers have plump or vesicular nuclei and sarcoplasmic basophilia due to increased RNA activity (Figure 1.5). Nuclei may become internalized.

Chronic myopathic processes are usually associated with a significant fiber size variation—with atrophy and hypertrophy—and myofibers tend to be rounded. Larger fibers may split. Fibrosis, an

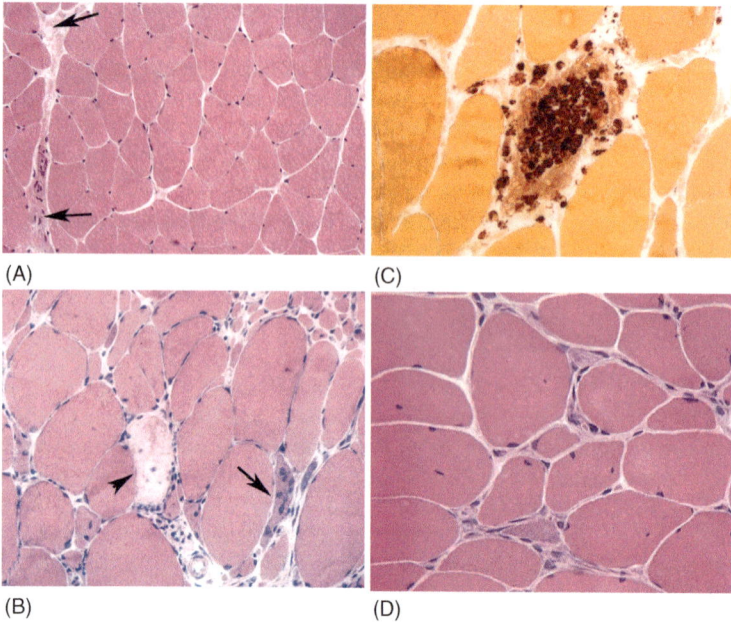

FIGURE 1.5 Normal muscle and basic histopathologic features of myopathy. (A) Normal muscle is shown. The arrows denote the perimysial connective tissue that divides fascicles. Individual myofibers are surrounded by endomysial connective tissue (Hematoxylin and eosin [H&E], frozen section]). (B) Myopathic changes include atrophic and hypertrophic fibers, consisting of a pale necrotic fiber (arrowhead) and a basophilic regenerating fiber containing enlarged nuclei (arrow) (H&E, frozen). (C) Macrophages are seen within a myofiber undergoing myophagocytosis (nonspecific esterase, frozen). (D) In this specimen from a patient with muscular dystrophy, there is an excess of endomysial connective tissue surrounding individual myofibers and several fibers with internalized nuclei.

increase in connective tissue, may develop along with fatty infiltration. These chronic myopathic changes are often said to have a *dystrophic* appearance histopathologically (Figure 1.5). However, not all muscular dystrophies exhibit such changes.

Differential Diagnosis of Myopathic Histopathology Findings
The differential diagnosis for the host of myopathic changes is broad and warrants additional histochemical and possibly immunohistochemical staining for metabolic disorders and potentially dystrophies or autoimmune processes. A list of commonly performed stains and description of their utility is found in Table 1.9.

For example, in *mitochondrial diseases*, *ragged red fibers* are usually seen with Gomori trichrome and fibers overreact with succinic dehydrogenase and may not react with cytochrome oxidase. Staining

TABLE 1.9 Histochemical Stains and Their Major Uses

Stain	Utility
• H&E	• Routine
• Gomori trichrome	• Mitochondria, rimmed vacuoles, rods, tubular aggregates
• NADH	• Myofibrillar changes (e.g., cores)
• ATPase	• Fiber typing, atrophy
• PAS	• Glycogen
• Oil-red-O or Sudan black	• Lipid
• Congo red	• Amyloid
• Cytochrome oxidase	• Mitochondria
• Succinic dehydrogenase	• Mitochondria
• Nonspecific esterase	• Denervation, macrophages
• Alkaline phosphatase	• Regeneration, connective tissue/dysimmune
• Acid phosphatase	• Macrophages • Lysosomes, autophagy
• Phosphorylase, PFK, MADA	• Metabolic disorders

ATPase, adenosine triphosphatase; H&E, hematoxylin and eosin; MADA, myoadenylate deaminase; NADH, nicotinamide adenine dehydrogenase; PAS, periodic acid schiff; PFK, phosphofructokinase.

for glycogen, lipid, and amyloid is easily performed on frozen tissue, and paraffin tissue can also be used for glycogen assessment. Histochemical staining for phosphorylase, phospho-fructokinase, and myoadenylate deaminase is also available.

Many immunostains are available for muscular dystrophies, but genetic testing is often necessary for diagnostic confirmation. Histochemical stains are also necessary to identify nemaline rods, cores, minicores, and tubular aggregates. Autophagic vacuoles may be highlighted with acid phosphatase. A list of stains performed on frozen tissue and description of their utility follows (Table 1.9):

- In *autoimmune myopathies,* there is usually lymphocytic inflammation.
- In *necrotizing autoimmune myopathy (NAIM),* there are mainly macrophages and few or no lymphocytes.
- In *dermatomyositis (DM),* there is usually perivascular, perimysial lymphocytic inflammation, accompanied by atrophy and degeneration of perifascicular fibers (Figure 1.6).

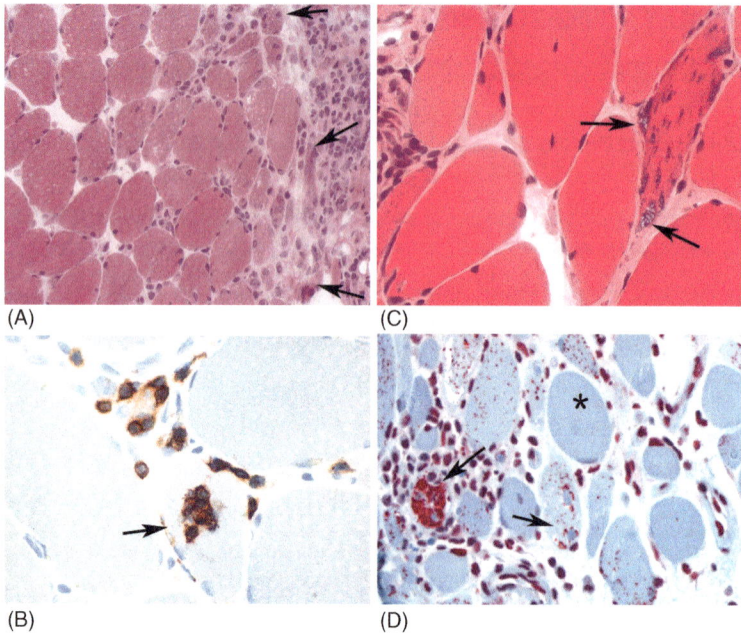

FIGURE 1.6 Inflammatory myopathies. **(A)** Dermatomyositis. One fascicle is shown with the arrows demarcating the edge (perifascicular region). There is atrophy of perifascicular myofibers, and perimysial lymphocytic inflammation is present at the back of the arrows (H&E, frozen). **(B)** Myofiber invasion is depicted. The myofiber in the center is not necrotic and is invaded by cytotoxic T cells (CD8 immunostain, frozen). **(C)** IBM. There are mononuclear inflammatory cells (upper left), hypertrophic and atrophic myofibers, and a fiber containing rimmed vacuoles (arrow). **(D)** IBM. A TDP-43 immunoreacted paraffin section is shown. TDP-43 is normally present in myofiber nuclei but not in the cytoplasm (the asterisk indicates a normal myofiber). In this specimen, the cytoplasm of many myofibers has TDP-43 reactive inclusions, and a large aggregate is denoted by the arrow.

H&E, hematoxylin and eosin; IBM, inclusion body myositis.

- In DM, antisynthetase syndrome, and some cases of NAIM, there is C5b-9 membrane attack complex (MAC) deposition in endomysial capillaries.

- In *polymyositis (PM)* and *inclusion body myositis (IBM)*, there tends to be predominant lymphocytic endomysial inflammation. Usually one can identify the presence of lymphocytes invading otherwise intact fibers (*myofiber invasion*; Figure 1.6).

- If immunohistochemistry is performed, these invading cells are usually cytotoxic T cells. Some perimysial inflammation is also common in these conditions.

- In IBM, there are usually features of a more chronic myopathy, along with the presence of "rimmed" vacuoles. Congo red–positive material may be seen in a minority of myofibers. Cytoplasmic conclusions may also immunoreact with a number of stains, including transactive DNA binding protein 43 (TDP43), p62 (sequestosome 1), and SMI 31 (phosphorylated neurofilament heavy; Figure 1.6).

Abnormal upregulation of major histocompatibility complex (MHC) class I on myofibers may be identified immunohistochemically. This finding is a useful and sensitive but nonspecific marker for an inflammatory myopathy. The presence of MHC II immunoreactivity is less sensitive but more specific for autoimmune processes.

In specimens in which there is inflammation without myofiber invasion, rimmed vacuoles, or perifascicular atrophy, and when the patient does not have clinical features of DM, the diagnosis of "nonspecific myositis" may be used, and all PM mimics should be considered such as IBM, dystrophies, and even metabolic disorders.

A summary of the histopathologic findings in autoimmune myopathies follows (Table 1.10).

Neurogenic Histopathologic Findings

- Neurogenic atrophy affects myofibers of both histochemical types (type 1 and type 2).
- The atrophic fibers are often angulated.
- There are usually associated nuclear clumps.
- Denervated fibers tend to stain darkly with nicotinamide adenine dinucleotide–tetrazolium reductase (NADH–TR) and nonspecific esterase.
- Target fibers, which are best seen with the NADH–TR reaction, have a bull's-eye type of appearance, and are pathognomonic of a neurogenic process (Figure 1.7).
- With *reinnervation*, there is loss of the normal checkerboard pattern of type 1 and type 2 muscle fibers intermingling. In addition, *fiber type grouping* occurs; it is seen best with the myosin adenosine triphosphatase (ATPase) stain.

Occasionally, there are mixed findings of a myopathic and neurogenic process. In some of these instances, myotonic dystrophies should come to mind as a diagnosis, especially if there are many internalized nuclei or ring fibers. Sometimes, myopathies such as myotonic dystrophy have a predominantly "neurogenic appearance." Chronic neurogenic processes such as spinal muscular atrophy type III may be associated with secondary myopathic changes; some chronic myopathies, such as IBM, also may have neurogenic features that are likely "secondary." Clinical and EMG correlation are paramount in diagnosing these conditions.

TABLE 1.10 Summary of Histopathologic Changes in Autoimmune Myopathies

Disorder	General	Inflammation	MHC 1	Other
Dermatomyositis	Perifascicular atrophy, myofiber degeneration and regeneration	Perimysial, CD4 > CD8 lymphocytes, B cells, macrophages, dendritic cells	Perifascicular predominant	Capillary microangiopathy (MAC deposition and capillary loss)
Polymyositis	Myofiber degeneration and regeneration, myofiber invasion	Endomysial > perimysial, CD8 > CD4 lympocytes	Endomysial, especially invaded fibers	
Inclusion body myositis	Chronic myopathic changes, rimmed vacuoles, myofiber invasion, mitochondrial changes	Endomysial CD8 > CD4; plasma cells	Endomysial, especially invaded fibers	Inclusions TDP-43, p62, SMI-31 and amyloid, EM: filamentous inclusions
Necrotizing autoimmune myopathy	Myofiber necrosis with myophagocytosis	Little or no lymphocytic inflammation	Variable	+/− MAC on capillaries

EM, electron microscopy; MAC, membrane attack complex; MHC1, major histocompatibility complex class I.

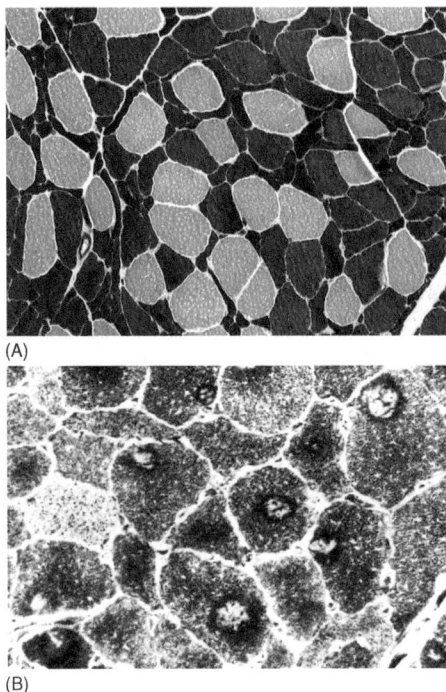

FIGURE 1.7 **(A) Atrophy exclusively involving the dark type 2 fibers is shown (ATPase, pH 9.4, frozen). (B) Neurogenic change. Target fibers are depicted. (NADH–TR, frozen).**

ATPase, adenosine triphosphatase; NADH–TR, nicotinamide adenine dinucleotide–tetrazolium reductase

Any process that causes denervation of muscle fibers can cause neurogenic changes, including axonal neuropathy with motor involvement, radiculopathy, anterior horn cell disorders, and even some primarily myopathic processes if the motor end-plate/muscle membrane region is affected.

Type 2 Myofiber Atrophy

Atrophy of only type 2 fibers should be distinguished from neurogenic atrophy (Figure 1.7). Neurogenic atrophy affects both type 1 and type 2 fibers, and some to many atrophic fibers that are overreactive with NADH–TR and esterase varies.

With type 2 fiber atrophy, the atrophic fibers are *not* overreactive with NADH–TR or esterase.

Type 2 fiber atrophy is nonspecific, but it is encountered with the following conditions:

- Corticosteroid use
- Disuse

- Connective tissue diseases in general
- Endocrinopathies
- NMJ disorders

The subtype of fibers that are atrophic are often the type 2b (fast glycolytic) fibers.

Nerve Biopsy
Introduction
In contrast to the evaluation of myopathy and the prominent role of muscle biopsy in its diagnosis, nerve biopsy is not a common component of the workup for PN. Usually, a sensory nerve, typically the superficial fibular/peroneal or sural nerve, is biopsied.

- The most common reason to biopsy a peripheral nerve is to evaluate the patient for suspected vasculitis. Concern about other inflammatory or infiltrative processes might be reasons for obtaining a biopsy as well.
- When vasculitis is suspected, a concomitant muscle biopsy may increase the diagnostic yield.

When interpreting the nerve biopsy report, just as with the muscle biopsy report, it is important to make a judgment as to whether the appropriate nerve was biopsied. In most instances, there should have been evidence of both clinical and electrophysiologic involvement of the biopsied nerve.

The most important preparation to be evaluated for inflammatory processes is the paraffin embedded section. However, in some laboratories, frozen sections are performed instead of paraffin embedding. Teased fibers are helpful, especially in assessing for demyelination. The 1-micron-thick, plastic (Epon)-embedded, thick (semithin) sections are very useful in visualizing the nerve morphology in greater detail compared to the paraffin sections (Figure 1.8). Those sections are then trimmed, cut thinner, placed on grids, stained with a heavy metal, and used for electron microscopy as needed.

Major Types of Nerve Pathology
Only a few major categories of histopathologic changes in peripheral nerves are distinguished:

- Axonal degeneration
- Demyelination
- Mixed axonal degeneration and demyelination

During the process of *axonal degeneration*, the axonal organelles are disturbed in some fashion within the intact myelin sheath, and such changes may be seen with electron microscopy. With light

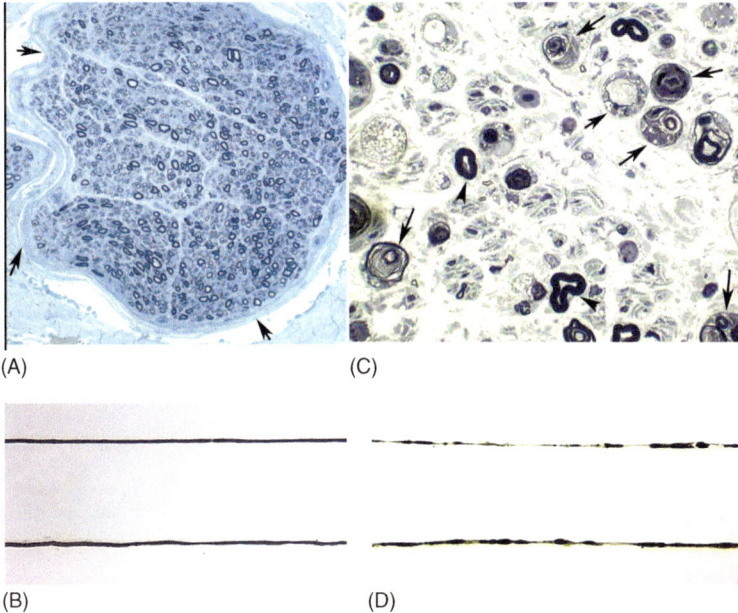

FIGURE 1.8 Normal nerve and axonal degeneration. (A) A normal nerve is shown, and the perineurium is designated by the arrows. The perineurium is the boundary of a fascicle (toluidine blue, plastic section). (B) Normal teased fibers. (C) Many myelin ovoids are shown in this nerve affected by vasculitis (see arrows for examples). A normal myelinated axon is depicted by the arrowhead (toluidine blue, plastic section). (D) Myelin ovoids (axonal degeneration) (teased fiber preparation).

microscopy, one sees retraction and collapse of the myelin sheath following axonal degeneration, and this retraction appears as a *myelin ovoid* (Figure 1.8). In cross section, the axon may appear to be expanded or ballooned with associated fragmentation of myelin. The debris is then engulfed by macrophages. Myelin ovoids are easily seen on teased fiber preparation as myelin fragmentation (Figure 1.8).

- In ischemic axonopathies, there may be variable, multifocal degeneration and loss of axons, as opposed to the more homogenous loss that might be expected in a "metabolic" disorder.
- Acute *demyelination* is difficult to evaluate on paraffin or frozen sections. On plastic-embedded, semithin sections and ultrastructural imaging, vesicular demyelination or splitting of the myelin sheath may be seen (Figure 1.9). These findings may be difficult to distinguish from artifact. Denuded axons may be seen on rare occasions.
- In autoimmune disorders, macrophages can sometimes be seen engulfing the myelin sheath. This process may need to be confirmed with electron microscopy.

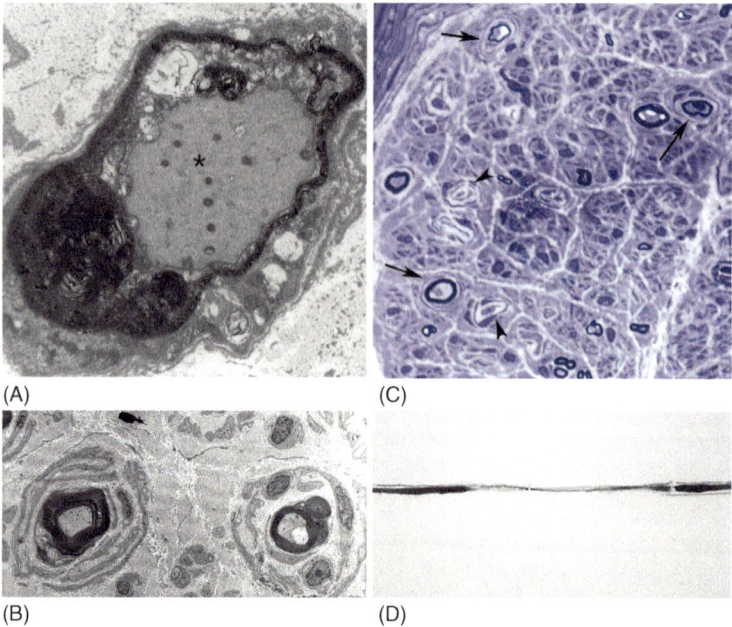

(A) (C)

(B) (D)

FIGURE 1.9 Demyelinating neuropathy. **(A)** Acute demyelination. The axon (*) is intact, but the myelin sheath is undergoing vesicular demyelination (electron photomicrograph). **(B)** There is loss of myelinated axons, and many onion bulbs are seen (see arrows for examples) (toluidine blue, plastic section). **(C)** Onion bulbs are seen via electron microscopy (CMT1). **(D)** The middle intermodal segment is undergoing demyelination (teased fiber preparation).

CMT1, Charcot-Marie-Tooth disease type 1.

- Teased fibers show evidence of segmental demyelination (Figure 1.9) as well as internodal segments—the regions between the nodes of Ranvier—of varying thickness and length, consistent with remyelination. Continued demyelination and remyelination manifest as *onion bulbs*, which can be seen to some degree on the paraffin sections, but are easiest to see on plastic-embedded sections and with electron microscopy (Figure 1.9).

With inflammatory disorders, lymphocytes may be seen in the endoneurium and around blood vessels in any of the nerve compartments (endoneurium, perineurium, and epineurium). Granulomas, which comprise loose collections of inflammatory cells including histiocytes, may be seen in sarcoidosis. Vasculitis affects epineurial blood vessels of various sizes (Figure 1.10).

Nerves should also be assessed for the presence of amyloid with stains such as Congo red, crystal violet, or thioflavin. Various lipid inclusions may be seen on semithick, plastic-embedded sections stained with toluidine blue in processes such as amiodarone and

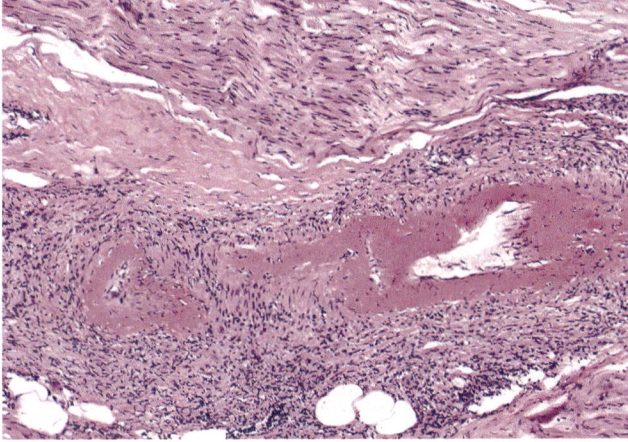

FIGURE 1.10 Vasculitic neuropathy. The large blood vessel at the bottom exhibits fibrinoid necrosis of the vessel wall with transmural inflammation (H&E paraffin).

H&E, hematoxylin and eosin.

hydroxychloroquine neurotoxicity and in storage diseases such as Fabry disease. The nature of these inclusions should be confirmed with ultrastructural study.

Histochemical staining for inflammatory cells subsets may be useful, especially if lymphoma is a consideration. Concomitant muscle biopsy, as mentioned earlier, is useful in evaluating patients for vasculitis since it increases the yield. It is also useful in the evaluation for amyloid.

A partial list of axonal and demyelinating neuropathies and their characteristic histopathologic findings follows (Tables 1.11 and 1.12).

TABLE 1.11 Axonal Neuropathies and Their Major Histopathologic Features

Neuropathy subtype	Key histopathologic features
Vasculitic	Transmural inflammation +/– fibrinoid necrosis of vessel walls; multifocal axonal degeneration
Diabetic	Mixed axonal degeneration and demyelination; blood vessel wall thickening; perineurial thickening and degeneration; occasionally neovascularization
Sarcoid	Granulomas; may have diffuse inflammation; axon loss

(*continued*)

TABLE 1.11 Axonal Neuropathies and Their Major Histopathologic Features (*continued*)

Neuropathy subtype	Key histopathologic features
CMT2	Usually nonspecific axonal degeneration and loss
Amyloid	Small > large nerve fibers involved; amyloid deposits in the endoneurium primarily
Storage diseases such as Fabry disease	May have complex lipid inclusions
Toxic (e.g., chemotherapeutic)	Axonal degeneration and loss; complex lipid inclusions with amiodarone, hydroxychloroquine and chloroquine
Lymphoma	B cells

CMT2, Charcot-Marie-Tooth disease type 2.

TABLE 1.12 Demyelinating Neuropathies and Their Major Histopathologic Features

Subtype	Other features
Acute inflammatory demyelinating	In some cases, endoneurial and perivascular lymphocytic inflammation; acute demyelination with myelin stripping by macrophages
Chronic inflammatory demyelinating	Lymphocytes in the endoneurium in about one-third; onion bulbs in many; thinly myelinated axons; axonal degeneration and loss
Paraproteinemia	Myelin sheath splitting in some; axon loss
CMT1	Onion bulbs; chronic axon loss
Amiodarone	Demyelination and axonal degeneration; lipid inclusions; may have vacuolar myopathy

CMT1, Charcot-Marie-Tooth disease type 1.

SUGGESTED READING

Ankala A, da Silva C, Gualandi F, et al. A comprehensive genomic approach for neuromuscular diseases gives a high diagnostic yield. *Ann Neurol.* 2015;77(2):206–214.

Daube JR, Rubin DI. Needle electromyography. *Muscle Nerve.* 2009;39:244–270.

Engel AG. *Myasthenia gravis and myasthenic disorders.* New York, NY: Oxford University Press; 1999.

England JD, Gronseth GS, Franklin G, et al. Evaluation of distal symmetric PN: the role of laboratory and genetic testing (an evidence-based review). *Muscle Nerve.* 2009;39(1):116–125.

Lacomis D. Electrodiagnostic approach to the patient with suspected myopathy. *Neurol Clin.* 2002:20;587–603.

Magri F, Nigro V, Angelini C, et al. The Italian limb girdle muscular dystrophy registry: relative frequency, clinical features, and differential diagnosis. *Muscle Nerve.* 2017;55(1):55–68. doi:10.1002/mus

Nojszewska M, Gawel M, Szmidt-Salkowska E, et al. Abnormal spontaneous activity in primary myopathic disorders. *Muscle Nerve.* 2016. doi: 10.1002/mus.25521. [Epub ahead of print]

Saporta AS, Sottile SL, Miller LJ, et al. Charcot-Marie-Tooth disease subtypes and genetic testing strategies. *Ann Neurol.* 2011;69(1):22–33.

Silvestri NJ, Wolfe GI. Asymptomatic/Pauci-symptomatic creatine kinase elevations (hyperCKemia). *Muscle Nerve.* 2013;47: 805–815.

Szczudlik P, Szyluk B, Lipowska M, et al. Antititin antibody in early- and late-onset myasthenia gravis. *Acta Neurol Scand.* 2014;130:229–233.

2 Acute Generalized Weakness

Simona Treidler and Yaacov Anziska

INTRODUCTION

Weakness is a common and nonspecific complaint that encompasses a broad differential diagnosis, including both neurologic and non-neurologic conditions. Weakness is broadly defined as the inability to perform a desired movement with normal force because of a reduction in muscle strength.

Normal motor function involves integrated muscle activity that is modulated by the entire neuro-axis, including the cerebral cortex, basal ganglia, cerebellum, spinal cord, nerve roots, peripheral nerves, neuromuscular junction, and muscle. The tempo of weakness onset, its distribution, and any accompanying symptoms help to determine its cause.

Weakness can be broadly categorized as focal or generalized.

- Generalized weakness, or quadriparesis, affects all extremities and results from either systemic disease (sepsis, cardiac failure, dehydration, severe hypokalemia, adrenal insufficiency), high spinal cord lesions, or certain neuromuscular disorders (myasthenia gravis [MG], Guillain-Barré syndrome [GBS], periodic paralysis). In generalized weakness, certain bulbar motor functions, such as facial movements, articulation, chewing, and swallowing, may also be involved.

- Focal weakness, by contrast, can result from spinal cord involvement or dysfunction of the peripheral nervous system. In spinal cord disease, the weakness is incomplete, with more severe involvement of muscles preferentially innervated by corticospinal tracts. Peripheral nerve disease tends to predominantly involve distal muscles, although there are exceptions. There is no preferential involvement of corticospinal tract–innervated muscles. In neuromuscular junction disorders and certain myopathies, the weakness is likely to be worse proximally, sensation is spared, reflexes are normal, and there is frequently involvement of bulbar muscles, especially with ptosis and ophthalmoplegia.

HISTORY

The most important element of the history of weakness is its time of onset; acute disease arises in minutes to hours (i.e., a vascular event), subacute disease emerges over weeks (e.g., GBS), and chronic disease endures for years (e.g., muscular dystrophy). Fluctuation of the weakness or presence of fatigability with sustained muscle effort suggests MG or a metabolic myopathy.

- Acute attacks of generalized weakness lasting for a few hours and spontaneously resolving are seen in periodic paralysis, as well as in transient vascular pathology. Repeated attacks of weakness suggest neuromuscular junction disorders, periodic paralysis, and metabolic myopathies.
- Another key element is the presence of an underlying neuromuscular disorder, which may worsen transiently, such as MG.
- A thorough history addresses certain medical comorbidities, such as renal failure, thyroid disease, and adrenal insufficiency.
- It is important to inquire about the patient's dietary habits and exposure to medications known to be myotoxic, such as statins.
- The examiner should not overlook use of illicit substances, such as cocaine, which can cause overwhelming rhabdomyolysis.
- The presence of preceding viral illnesses and vaccinations suggest a viral myositis or GBS, and history of recent travel could implicate a tick paralysis or an acute generalized neuropathy (acute motor axonal neuropathy, GBS).
- Family history is typically more important when diagnosing chronic weakness, such as muscular dystrophy. In rare cases, a positive history can aid in diagnosing subtler causes of weakness, including metabolic myopathy and periodic paralysis.

SIGNS

Quadriparesis

- Quadriparesis, or weakness of all limbs, when associated with impairment of mental status, is a sign of a diffuse cerebral process such as anoxia, severe hypotension, cerebral edema from head trauma, or systemic metabolic abnormalities.
- Quadriparesis with upper motor neuron signs (weakness of upper limb extensors and lower limb flexors, hyperreflexia, and extensor plantar reflex) and cranial nerve deficits (dysarthria, dysphagia, ophthalmoplegia) is usually associated with a brainstem lesion, and a rapid diagnosis is essential for possible surgical management. Table 2.1 distinguishes signs and symptoms due to upper versus lower motor neuron lesions. Association of quadriparesis with a sensory level and bowel or bladder abnormalities localizes the lesion to the cervical spine. This etiology can be life threatening, as

TABLE 2.1 Upper Versus Lower Motor Neuron Weakness

Feature	Upper motor neuron	Lower motor neuron
Weakness distribution	Corticospinal distribution (extensors in upper limbs and flexors in lower limbs)	Generalized proximal/distal with no preferential involvement
Sensory involvement	Central pattern	None/root/ stocking-glove/nerve distributions
Deep tendon reflexes	Decreased/increased	Normal/decreased
Pathologic reflexes	Present	Absent
Sphincter function	Could be impaired	Normal/impaired in cauda equina lesion
Muscle tone	Increased/normal or decreased in acute process	Normal/decreased
Muscle bulk	Normal/slight atrophy due to disuse	Atrophy may be marked
Fasciculations	No	Possible

it may impair the diaphragmatic ventilatory function and disrupt the autonomic nervous system, leading to hypotension and tachycardia.

- The presence of quadriparesis with lower motor neuron signs (flaccid tone, diminished or absent reflexes, +/– fasciculations) with sensory abnormalities is most consistent with an acute polyneuropathy, such as GBS, also leading to ventilatory failure. The absence of sensory symptoms points to a myositis, as most myopathies do not present acutely.

- Quadripareis presenting with ocular (diplopia, ptosis) and bulbar weakness (dysarthria, dysphagia) usually occurs in a neuromuscular junction disorder (MG, Lambert-Eaton myasthenic syndrome [LEMS]), as this kind of disorder can also cause respiratory failure.

- Quadriparesis can be associated with other patterns of weakness, including disproportionate proximal or distal weakness, axial weakness, and bulbar, ocular, or facial dysfunction.

Proximal Weakness

- Proximal weakness, including bibrachial palsy and flail arm syndrome, can be seen in the early stages of GBS and in motor neuropathies resulting from amyloidosis or porphyria. Yet, "man in the barrel syndrome" can also be caused by bilateral watershed brain infarcts. A central cervical spinal cord lesion produces the same pattern of weakness, but there is usually loss of pain and temperature sensation in the arms. While proximal weakness is more characteristic in autoimmune myositis, other myopathies, such as metabolic, endocrine, and toxic forms, can be responsible, though rarely in the acute setting. MG can first present with acute proximal weakness and progress to generalized weakness, usually over a period of days. An adult form of acid maltase deficiency and familial periodic paralysis may affect only the proximal muscles.

Distal Weakness

- Distal weakness rarely generalizes acutely, except in GBS and central cord syndrome. Patients will complain of difficulty climbing onto a sidewalk due to foot drop. As the disease progresses, they will have difficulty buttoning a shirt, using a zipper, and opening a jar. If the physical exam reveals weakness and dissociated loss of pain and temperature, then a central cord process is more likely. If there is weakness and areflexia, then GBS is the usual culprit.

Facial and Bulbar Weakness

- Facial and bulbar weakness can be associated with generalized weakness in neuromuscular junction disorders (botulism, MG), GBS, and brainstem strokes. Patients will complain of difficulty drinking through a straw, and lower facial weakness will produce drooling and difficulty handling saliva. Weakness of masticatory muscles, as in MG, may cause fatigue and difficulty chewing. Pharyngeal, palatal, and tongue weakness disturb speech and swallowing. A flaccid palate is associated with nasal regurgitation, choking, and aspiration of liquids. Speech becomes slurred or acquires a nasal or hoarse quality.

Neck Weakness

- Neck weakness occurs in many neuromuscular conditions, including polymyositis, motor neuron disease (MND), and MG. Patients can suffer either from neck flexor or extensor weakness; in the latter, they will have the "dropped head" syndrome. Examination of neck strength in acute muscle weakness is a crude test of respiratory impairment, as these muscles and the diaphragm may be simultaneously affected by similar processes. Shortness of breath is typically reported when prone. Since diaphragmatic weakness leads to hypoventilation and carbon dioxide retention, patients may complain of morning headaches, and in the later stages of hypercapnia, may become lethargic or confused. Acute onset of shortness of breath occurs in acute motor neuropathies, MG, myositis, and high cervical transverse myelitis.

Paraparesis/Paraplegia

- Paraparesis, paraplegia, or symmetric weakness of the legs, with or without an accompanying sensory level, is generally caused by a spinal cord lesion at or below the upper thoracic spinal cord.

- Paraparesis can also result from lesions at other locations that disturb both upper motor neurons (i.e., parasagittal tumors and strokes) and lower motor neurons (such as MND, cauda equina syndrome, and peripheral neuropathies).
- Acute paraplegia at an early stage can be associated with flaccid tone and absent reflexes, making localization to the spinal cord challenging. Alternatively, it could be consistent with a rapidly progressive MND (polio, West Nile virus) or with GBS.
- The presence of a thoracic sensory level and increased reflexes in the lower limbs should guide the examiner to consider a thoracic cord process, such as an epidural tumor, abscess, hematoma, prolapsed disc, spinal cord infarction (sparing proprioception), arteriovenous fistula, and transverse myelitis.

PHYSICAL EXAMINATION OF A WEAK PATIENT
General Physical Examination

- A general examination should be performed before focusing on the neurologic exam. Special attention should be directed to any signs of chronic systemic illness, occult neoplasms, chronic infections, or endocrine dysfunction. An important component of this examination is the recognition of life-threatening respiratory failure or cardiac arrhythmias, so as to decide on admission to a monitored setting, possible intubation, and initiation of anti-arrhythmic medications.
- Unlike those individuals with respiratory failure associated with primary cardiac or respiratory disorders, patients with neuromuscular conditions and significant respiratory dysfunction can appear asymptomatic, without typical signs (such as use of accessory muscles, shallow breathing, or wheezing) until they finally decompensate with disease progression. Respiratory function should always be evaluated in *all* patients with generalized neuromuscular weakness.

Respiratory Pattern

- The pattern of respiratory muscle function is helpful for making a diagnosis. At rest, diaphragmatic movement performs the majority of ventilatory function. Patients with isolated diaphragmatic weakness compensate during inspiration by using the accessory muscles of respiration (pectoral, scalene, intercostal, and sternocleidomastoid muscles).
- Diaphragmatic paralysis can be observed by "paradoxical" abdominal movement, with inward movement of the abdominal wall on inspiration. In contrast, patients with impaired intercostal muscle function and preserved diaphragmatic function exhibit inward movement of the upper ribcage and intercostal spaces during inspiration. Auscultation of the chest is often unremarkable

in these patients, although crepitations may be heard, reflecting atelectasis. On rare occasions, transmitted upper airway sounds may be present in patients with bulbar dysfunction.

Bedside Testing

- The "single breath" counting test performed at the bedside tests the ability to count after a maximal inspiration. Patients with a normal respiratory function can reach up to 50, and anything less than 15 correlates with severe impairment of vital capacity. Laborious breathing while lying flat is another important indication of diaphragmatic weakness and reduced vital capacity, causing orthopnea.

- Bedside spirometry is critical for measurement of ventilatory function in those with neuromuscular disorders, especially in the acute setting. Respiratory thresholds are remembered best through the *"20/30/40 rule,"* applicable to standard spirometry assessment. Significant ventilatory dysfunction is reflected by forced vital capacity (FVC) less than 20 mL/kg, maximal inspiratory pressure (MIP) of 30 cm H_2O or less, and maximal expiratory pressure (MEP) less than 40 cm H_2O; any abnormal values should trigger critical care support. The objective of bedside spirometry is to detect emerging hypoventilation prior to life-threatening decompensation culminating in hypoxemia, which is detectable by pulse oximetry or arterial blood gas measurement. However, checking pulse oximetry and/or blood gases earlier in the disease course may falsely reassure the examiner, as these will remain normal until there is significant disease progression.

- Dysarthria, presence of a weak cough with difficulty clearing secretions, "staccato speech," and hypophonia are other important signs of bulbar and respiratory dysfunction that are noted at the bedside. Difficulty lifting the head against gravity correlates with significant diaphragmatic weakness, as both of these areas share similar nerve root innervation.

- Autonomic dysfunction is common in patients with acute neuromuscular diseases, occurring in up to 60% of cases of GBS. Clinical manifestations include orthostatic hypotension, diabetes insipidus, ileus, and cardiac arrhythmias. All of these conditions may require medical treatment, occasionally even emergency pacing. Bedside assessment of blood pressure (supine and sitting) *and* a standard EKG are part of the initial evaluation.

The Neurologic Examination

The neurologic examination, with careful attention to strength testing, sensory modalities, and deep tendon reflexes, is necessary in all patients who complain of acute weakness. In situations that suggest a central process or an ascending paralysis, a detailed evaluation of the cranial nerves should be performed, in addition to the motor and sensory examination.

The goals of the neurologic examination are as follows:

1. Clarify the exact nature of the clinical symptoms. Is the patient truly weak?
2. Identify clinical symptoms not recognized by the patient. For example, is weakness of the legs accompanied by mild, but less evident, weakness in the arms? Is the weakness accompanied by sensory loss not recognized by the patient?
3. Clarify the anatomic basis for the symptoms. Is the weakness accompanied by changes in the deep tendon reflexes, or by muscle atrophy and fasciculations? Table 2.2 provides a concise guide to aid in lesion localization. Table 2.3 reviews localization in lesions of the peripheral nervous system.

- First, the examiner must inspect the various muscles, looking for atrophy or hypertrophy, as well as spontaneous involuntary movements, including fasciculations, muscle "rippling," and myokymias. While muscle strength evaluation is commonly regarded as "objective," as it is rated on a numerical scale, this assessment is actually quite subjective and is highly dependent on the skill of the physician. It is also important that the patient exerts a maximum effort. It can be difficult to assess strength reliably in an individual with severe pain or an individual who is unwilling to fully cooperate with the examination. Patients with anxiety or depression may not be motivated to make a full effort on strength testing.
- Peripheral nerve hypertrophy is seen and/or felt in certain demyelinating polyneuropathies, including hereditary motor-sensory neuropathy, leprosy, and neurofibromatosis.
- In the acute setting, the most important causes of acute generalized weakness without localizing signs are disorders affecting the peripheral nerves, the neuromuscular junction, and the muscles. Their clinical features can help differentiate them.

DIAGNOSTIC INVESTIGATIONS

- The extent of diagnostic testing performed on a weak patient varies depending on the differential diagnosis and the potential rate of clinical deterioration. A patient with severe sepsis will need a full workup to identify the source and subsequent treatment. If one suspects an acute stroke or spinal cord lesion, the following tests should be performed emergently.

Imaging

1. Computed tomography (CT) of head and/or CT angiography head and neck for evaluation of a central lesion.
2. Magnetic resonance imaging (MRI) of the spine (or CT myelography when MRI is contraindicated) for evaluation of spine lesions.

TABLE 2.2 Lesion Localization

Location	Weakness	Sensory loss	Deep tendon reflexes	Other features
Cerebral cortex	UMN pattern	Higher order	Increased	Loss of higher cognitive functions, seizures
Cerebral white matter and subcortical structures	UMN pattern	Higher order (cerebrum) Lower order (thalamus)	Increased	Loss of higher cognitive functions, psychiatric disturbances, movement disorders
Brainstem	UMN pattern	Lower order	Increased	Cranial nerve dysfunction contralateral to long-tract abnormality
Spinal cord	UMN below lesion LMN at the lesion level	Lower order	Increased	Sensory level at or below lesion; bowel/bladder dysfunction
Peripheral nerve	LMN pattern	Lower order	Decreased	Root or nerve distribution of the deficit
Neuro-muscular junction	Myopathic	None	Normal	Fatigable weakness of proximal or bulbar muscles
Muscle	Myopathic	None	Normal	Nonfatigable weakness of proximal muscles

LMN, lower motor neuron; UMN, upper motor neuron. Myopathic (diffuse, proximal weakness); higher order (stereognosia, two-point discrimination); lower order (modalities such as light touch, temperature).

Routine Laboratory Tests

1. Comprehensive metabolic panel and electrolytes. Elevated liver enzymes (aspartate transaminase [AST], alanine transaminase [ALT]) could indicate acute muscle destruction, such as in a myositis, but would not be accompanied by an elevated gamma-glutamyl transferase (GGT) level as in liver failure.

TABLE 2.3 Generalized Weakness: Peripheral Localization

Clinical signs	Neuropathy	Neuromuscular junction	Myopathy
Weakness pattern	Distal > proximal	Variable	Proximal > distal
Weakness severity	Constant, progressive	Variable	Constant, progressive
Sensory loss	Distal > proximal	Absent	Absent
Pain	Variable, distal	Absent	Usually absent
Muscle atrophy	Variable, often early	Absent	Variable, usually late
Reflexes	Decreased or absent	Normal	Normal or slightly decreased
Fasciculations	Sometimes	Absent	Absent
CSF	Normal or increased	Normal	Normal
CK	Normal or minimally increase	Normal	Increased
Edophronium test	No response	May respond	No response

CK, creatine kinase; CSF, cerebrospinal fluid.

- Hypokalemia or hyperkalemia is frequently seen in patients with periodic paralysis who experience transient and recurrent generalized muscle weakness. Hypokalemia, which can cause a myopathy, is also present in patients with renal disorders, such as renal tubular acidosis types 1 and 2, as well as in those using diuretics, laxatives, and glucocorticoids.
- Various metabolic derangements can cause generalized weakness, including hyponatremia or hypernatremia (seen in syndrome of inappropriate antidiuretic hormone secretion [SIADH], diabetes insipidus), hypercalcemia, and uremia.
2. Serum creatine kinase (CK). This test is valuable for evaluation of patients with neuromuscular disease. Although it is a marker of muscle disease, increased serum CK can be seen in MND and other neurogenic disorders. Conversely, elevated CK levels do not occur in all myopathies. The level of CK does not appear to correlate with the degree of muscle destruction or weakness. In normal individuals, levels may reach 5 times the upper limit of normal in certain situations, such as after an electrodiagnostic studies, and can be as high as 50 times the upper limit of normal

after extreme and prolonged exercise. Other muscle enzymes, including LDH and aldolase, should be also sent.

3. TSH, PTH, vitamin D, and cortisol levels for treatable causes of generalized weakness.

4. Vitamin B levels (B_1, B_6, B_{12}), vitamin E, and folic acid, which if abnormal, can cause neuropathy, myelopathy, or myopathy.

5. In the setting of a suspected myositis, one should order anti-nuclear antibody (ANA), double-stranded deoxyribonucleic acid (ds-DNA), anti-neutrophil cytoplasmic antibody (ANCA), cryoglobulins, rheumatoid factor, anti-Sjögren's syndrome A (anti-SSA), anti-Sjögren's syndrome B (anti-SSB), and angiotensin converting enzyme (ACE).

6. Infectious tests for generalized weakness, including HIV, human T-lymphotropic virus types 1 and 2 (HTLV-1/2), and hepatitis B and C serologies, along with Lyme disease (Western blotting). *Clostridium botulinum* toxin can be detected in blood or stool, especially in the presentation of acute descending weakness accompanied by cranial nerve and parasympathetic dysfunction and rapid respiratory failure.

7. Acetylcholine receptor (binding, blocking, modulating), muscle-specific kinase (MuSK), LRP4, agrin, and anti-voltage-gated calcium-channel antibodies to diagnose a neuromuscular junction disease.

8. Urine porphyrin (uroporphyrin, coproporphyrin), delta amino-levulinic acid, and porphobilinogen (sensitive and specific in an acute attack) could be obtained from urine for porphyric neuropathies.

9. Serum heavy metal testing, including arsenic, lead, mercury, and thalium, in the setting of a motor neuropathy.

Other Monitoring

1. EKG/cardiac monitoring, as generalized weakness can be a feature of acute myocardial infarction or exacerbation of cardiac failure. Cardiac arrhythmias are present in electrolyte abnormalities associated with generalized weakness and in channelopathies.

2. Chest x-ray can show a low-seated diaphragm, cardiomegaly, or pleural effusions.

3. Cerebrospinal fluid (CSF) analysis is indicated in suspected GBS, focusing on the albumino-cytologic dissociation, with elevated protein level and absent white blood cell count. However, detection of an elevated protein level is dependent on the timing of the lumbar puncture. The presence of lymphocytosis may be indicative of HIV infection or lymphoma and needs further evaluation. Bacterial, viral, and fungal cultures, along with tuberculosis

amplification via polymerase chain reaction (PCR), are important in the initial evaluation of an acute neuropathy, myopathy, or myelopathy.
4. Nerve conduction studies (NCS)/electromyography (EMG) are rarely used in the acute evaluation of generalized weakness.

In GBS, NCS may show prolonged or absent F waves, and rarely conduction block. EMG showing spontaneous activity suggests an acute inflammatory myositis.

DIFFERENTIAL DIAGNOSIS
A myriad of medical and neurologic disorders manifest with generalized weakness. This section focuses on the most common disorders of the peripheral nervous system presenting as acute generalized weakness.

Guillain-Barré Syndrome
- GBS is an immune-mediated neuropathy that presents with acute generalized weakness. Typically demyelinating, GBS is frequently preceded by infections, such as *Campylobacter jejuni*, or even by vaccinations, such as influenza. The suspected pathophysiology is molecular mimicry between *C. jejuni* lipooligosaccharides and GM1 or GD1a gangliosides at the nodes of Ranvier; GM1 and GD1a antibodies bind to these saccharides and activate the myelin-destroying complement apparatus. Table 2.4 provides a differential diagnosis of acute generalized weakness.
- GBS progresses within 1 to 2 weeks, first characterized by severe back pain and limb paresthesias, followed by ascending weakness, where proximal weakness exceeds distal weakness, and depressed/absent deep tendon reflexes. Facial and oropharyngeal muscles are affected in 50% of patients and can sometimes be the initial manifestation.
- Variants of GBS include Miller Fisher syndrome (ophthalmoplegia, ataxia, and areflexia), isolated paraparesis, pharyngeal–cervical–brachial weakness +/- ataxia, and bifacial weakness +/- distal paresthesias.
- Respiratory failure is the most dangerous complication of GBS, as it can lead to low tidal volume and poor gas exchange, resulting in hypercapnia. Another worrisome complication is dysautonomia, characterized by blood pressure fluctuations, cardiac arrhythmias, and gastrointestinal/bladder dysfunction. A few disorders mimic GBS, including transverse myelitis, MG, botulism, and carcinomatous or lymphomatous meningitis.
- CSF analysis typically reveals an elevated protein level with a normal white blood cell count. More than 10 lymphocytes/mm^3 could

TABLE 2.4 Differential Diagnosis of Acute Weakness

Systemic Causes
Sepsis
Severe anemia
Heart failure
Hepatic failure
Acute kidney injury
Hypoxemia/anoxic injury/hypercarbia
Hypoglycemia/hyperglycemia/hyperosmolar state
Electrolyte abnormalities (hypo/hyperkalemia, hypo/hypernatremia, hypo/hypercalcemia, hypermagnesemia, hypophosphatemia)
Thyroid dysfunction (hyperthyroid storm, myxedema)
Adrenal dysfunction (hyperaldosteronism/hypercortisolism/adrenal insufficiency)
Hypothermia/hyperthermia
Neuroleptic malignant syndrome
Malignant hyperthermia
Intoxications (alcohol/opiates/barbiturates/antidepressants/antipsychotic/anticonvulsants/illicit drugs)

Central Nervous System Disorders
Acute ischemic strokes (bilateral anterior cerebral artery (ACA) strokes, watershed infarcts, thalamic or brainstem)
Hemorrhagic strokes (large with midline shift or herniation)
Parasagittal frontal tumors
Syringobulbia
Infections: meningitis/encephalitis
Nonconvulsive status epilepticus
Postictal paralysis
Migraine with brainstem aura
Neuroinflammatory disorders (multiple sclerosis/neuromyelitis optica/acute disseminated encephalomyelitis, sarcoidosis, rheumatoid arthritis, systemic lupus erythematosus [SLE])
Severe Parkinson disease or Parkinsonian syndrome
Stiff person syndrome

Spinal Cord Disorders
Transverse myelitis
Syringomyelia
Neuroinflammatory disorders (multiple sclerosis/neuromyelitis optica/acute disseminated encephalomyelitis, sarcoidosis, rheumatoid arthritis, SLE)
Human immunodeficiency virus (HIV), human T-lymphotropic virus types 1 and 2 (HTLV-1/2), West Nile myelopathy
Subacute combined degeneration
Tabes dorsalis
Spinal cord infarction
Spinal cord compression (trauma/tumor/abscess/hemorrhage)

(*continued*)

TABLE 2.4 Differential Diagnosis of Acute Weakness (*continued*)

Peripheral Nerve Disorders
Toxic neuropathies (heavy metals, drugs, alcohol, and organophosphates)
Infectious neuropathies (HIV, cytomegalovirus [CMV], Epstein-Barr virus
[EBV], Lyme disease, HIV)
Acute inflammatory demyelinating polyneuropathy (Guillain-Barré
syndrome [GBS] and variants)
Thiamine deficiency
Vitamin B_{12} deficiency
Hypothyroid neuropathy
Diabetes neuropathies
Uremic neuropathy
Porphyria
Critical illness polyneuropathy

Neuromuscular Junction Disorders
Myasthenia gravis
Eaton-Lambert syndrome
Tetanus
Botulism
Tick paralysis
Insect/marine toxins

Myopathies
Polymyositis
Dermatomyositis
Necrotizing myopathy
Periodic paralysis
Alcohol myopathy
Medication-induced myopathies

Other Causes of Weakness
Motor neuron disease
Polyomyelitis

be seen in Lyme disease, HIV, poliomyelitis, West Nile virus, sarcoid disease, and leptomeningeal disease. CSF could be normal in the early presentation, as can the NCS, and there may not be absent F waves, prolonged distal latencies, decreased conduction velocities, or conduction block; there is typically sural nerve sparing.

- Bedside pulmonary function tests (maximal expiratory pressure [MEP] and maximal inspiratory pressure [MIP]) are invaluable, as those patients with diaphragmatic weakness will have a decrease in the forced vital capacity (FVC) when supine, with a 25% reduction from the baseline.
- Immunotherapy hastens recovery and decreases the risk of intubation by 50%. Intravenous immunoglobulins (IVIG) 0.4 g/kg/day for 5 days are the first-line treatment, due to availability and ease of administration. Potential mechanisms of action include

modulation of pathogenic autoantibody production, inhibition of antibodies, Fc receptor blockade, and immunoregulation of B and T cells. Plasma exchange is another treatment that removes antibodies and treats GBS, usually after five courses of plasma exchange.

- Overall mortality due to adult respiratory distress syndrome, sepsis, or dysautonomia is 3% to 5%, and those patients requiring mechanical ventilation have a 20% mortality rate. Only 79% of survivors can walk independently at 1 year, with severe disability occurring in 10% to 15% of GBS cases.

Myasthenia Gravis

- MG is an autoimmune disease in which antibodies bind to acetylcholine receptors or to similar molecules in the postsynaptic membrane at the neuromuscular junction. The antibody attack on the neuromuscular junction leads to weakness of skeletal muscles, whether generalized or ocular, and is more proximal than distal in presentation.

- Ocular MG (OMG) presents with fluctuating diplopia and ptosis. Bulbar muscles may also be involved, causing dysarthria or dysphagia. There may be weakness of neck flexors and/or extensors, and all weakness (generalized or ocular) typically worsens with exercise and fluctuates over the course of the day. MG should be considered in any patient who present with sudden weakness, especially if it fluctuates.

- The diagnosis of MG is confirmed by a combination of relevant symptoms and signs and a positive test for specific autoantibodies, including acetylcholine receptors, muscle-specific kinase (MuSK), and lipoprotein receptor–related protein 4 (LRP4). These antibodies are quite sensitive and specific. In seronegative cases, neurophysiological testing, along with repetitive nerve stimulation and single-fiber EMG, may be necessary for disease confirmation. While some have used the "edrophonium test" or infusion of short-acting edrophonium chloride, this diagnostic test lacks both sensitivity and specificity, as well as requiring cardiac monitoring.

- Myasthenia crisis is a life-threatening situation defined as respiratory failure due to severe diaphragmatic weakness, requiring intubation, especially if the vital capacity is less than 15 mL/kg or MIP is less than 15 to 20 mm H_2O. Severe bulbar weakness with inability to adequately protect the airways is another presentation of a crisis. Mortality in myasthenic crises ranges from 4% to 10%.

- Treatment of crisis first requires addressing the underlying cause for exacerbation, such as infection or medications worsening neuromuscular transmission (i.e., aminoglycosides, macrolides, and antiarrhythmics).

- In the acute setting, one can use either plasmapheresis (which directly removes antibodies from the peripheral circulation) or intravenous immunoglobulin, at 2 g/kg total over 5 days. Maintenance therapy with an immunomodulator, such as steroids, should be started. Steroids work fastest, but there are numerous other possibilities. Table 2.5 provides a list of disorders of the neuromuscular junction other than myasthenia.

Botulism

- Botulism is a rare cause of acute muscle weakness. It is caused by an exotoxin of *Clostridium botulinum*, an anaerobic bacterium that may contaminate improperly preserved or prepared food. The toxin acts at the neuromuscular junction to prevent the release of acetylcholine, thereby blocking neuromuscular transmission.

- Clinical symptoms usually appear 12 to 36 hours after the ingestion of contaminated food. The initial symptoms are typically related to impaired gastrointestinal motility (constipation, emesis, and abdominal cramps), followed by neurologic symptoms involving the extraocular, facial, and pharyngeal muscles. There may be ptosis, "blurred" vision, diplopia, facial weakness, dysarthria, dysphagia, and hoarseness. These early symptoms are similar to those seen in MG, except that in botulism, the pupillary reflexes are affected early. The weakness spreads rapidly to the muscles of the trunk and extremities and may progress to complete quadriplegia. As the weakness progresses, it can mimic GBS, but there are no sensory symptoms, and deep

---

TABLE 2.5 Causes of Neuromuscular Transmission Disorders Other Than Myasthenia Gravis

Presynaptic
LEMS
Botulism
Tick paralysis
Congenital myasthenia gravis
Toxins: elapid snakes species, arhropodes, marine species
Drugs: aminoglycosides, calcium-channel blockers, aminopyridines, corticosteroids
Synaptic
Congenital myasthenic syndromes
Drugs: reversible/irreversible cholinesterase inhibitors (edrophonium, pyridostigmine, organophosphates, and carbamates)
Postsynaptic
Drug-induced myasthenia gravis: penicillamine, alpha interferon
Congenital myasthenic syndromes
Drugs and toxins: nondepolarizing/depolarizing blocking agents
Antibiotics: tetracycline

LEMS, Lambert-Eaton myasthenic syndrome.

tendon reflexes are preserved. Careful observation suggests that ventilatory muscle weakness precedes the recognition of limb weakness.

- Respiratory failure is the most common cause of death and can occur within 6 to 8 hours of the onset of symptoms. Diagnosis includes demonstration of botulinum toxin in serum, in stool, or in food that the patient has recently consumed. Treatment consists of administration of heptavalent antitoxin as soon as possible. Pyridostigmine and 3,4-diaminopyridine may be used for symptomatic relief.

Organophosphate Compounds

- Organophosphate compounds are widely used as insecticides and more rarely in chemical warfare. These agents inhibit acetylcholinesterase, acting as cholinergic agents. Symptoms of acute poisoning develop immediately after the exposure and include nausea, vomiting, abdominal cramps, diarrhea, increased salivation, lacrimation, bronchospasm, and diffuse muscle weakness. Death results from respiratory failure, although treatment with pralidoxime can reverse the effects if administered within 24 to 48 hours. Atropine will reverse only the effects of excessive cholinergic stimulation on muscarinic receptors; it does not reverse the muscle weakness that results from overstimulation of nicotinic receptors.
  Other neurotoxins are presented in Table 2.6.

Disorders of Muscle

- Acute necrosis of muscle cells (rhabdomyolysis) liberates myoglobin, and high concentrations can cause acute renal failure. The most common causes are either toxic/drug-induced or physical (status epilepticus, trauma, or prolonged immobility) conditions. In rare cases, rhabdomyolysis can be the presenting sign of underlying muscle diseases, such as glycogen storage disorders.

Rhabdomyolysis

- Rhabdomyolysis can also result from myositis, or inflammation of the muscles. Myositis can be caused by infections (viral, bacterial, fungal, or parasitic), or drugs/toxins, electrolyte abnormalities (potassium, calcium), or it can be idiopathic (polymyositis, dermatomyositis, necrotizing myopathy). Table 2.7 provides a list of myotoxic drugs.

- The clinical presentation consists of proximal muscle weakness with or without myalgias. In the idiopathic forms, there may be associated lung, skin, and cardiac involvement. Laboratory testing demonstrates elevated muscle enzymes, presence of specific autoantibodies, and characteristic muscle biopsy changes.

- Treatment is directed at stopping exposure to the toxic agent, providing ventilator support, and avoiding metabolic disturbances by

TABLE 2.6 Neurotoxic Substances

Heavy Metals
Arsenic
Lead
Gold
Thallium
Mercury
Chemical Compounds
Organophosphates
Plants and Animal Toxins
Ciguatera
Paralytic shellfish poisoning
Puffer fish
Medications
Isoniazid
Ethambutol
Chloramphenicol
Linezolide
Dapsone
Fluoroquinolones
Pyridoxine
Nitrous oxide
Tacrolimus
Colchicine
Disulfiram
Procainamide
Amiodarone
Antiretroviral agents
Antineoplastic Agents
Vinka alkaloids
Platinum-containing drugs
Etoposide
Suramin
Ifosfamide
Thalidomide
Bortezomib

TABLE 2.7 Medications Causing Myopathy

Steroids
Colchicine
Zidovudine, other anti-HIV-related retroviral medications
Chloroquine/hydroxychloroquine
Amiodarone
Cholesterol-lowering (statins > fibrates, niacin, ezetimibe)
Proprofol
Cyclosporine
Tacrolimus
Imatinib
Amphotericin

aggressive hydration and electrolyte correction. Immediate treatment with pulse steroids is required for the idiopathic myositis entities.

Periodic Paralysis

- Periodic paralysis and other metabolic abnormalities can manifest clinically as generalized weakness. Periodic paralysis disorders are channelopathies caused by mutations of the genes controlling the structure of various channels (sodium, calcium, and chloride). The symptoms are triggered by stress, high-carbohydrate meals, extreme temperature, and heavy exercise.
- Hypokalemic periodic paralysis has two presentations. The autosomal dominant disorder is due to a defect in the muscle membrane's calcium or sodium channels, whereas the thyrotoxic periodic paralysis occurs in association with hyperthyroidism.
  - The clinical presentation most often first occurs in the teenage years, with generalized weakness and preserved consciousness lasting hours to days. Patients may awaken paralyzed after engaging in strenuous exercise or having eaten a meal rich in carbohydrates the night before. There is sparing of muscles of the face and trunk, and deep tendon reflexes are diminished or lost, but sensory examination is normal.
  - Diagnosis is based on suspicion, presence of repeated similar episodes in patient history, positive family history, and abnormal potassium level noted on testing. As untreated attacks last longer, potassium should be administered in the acute setting. Thyroid function testing should also be performed during the evaluation of a patient with such acute and diffuse muscle weakness.
- Hyperkalemic periodic paralysis is rarer, and the genetic defect occurs in the sodium channel. The clinical attacks are briefer and occur after exercise or ingestion of meals rich in potassium. The cranial and trunk muscles are not usually involved, and the attacks mostly resolve before patients arrive in the emergency department. In severe situations, administration of intravenous calcium gluconate, glucose, insulin, or beta-2 agonists can alleviate the attacks.

ICU-Acquired Weakness

- Flaccid paralysis of the limbs may develop in patients in critical care units, typically within a week, but sometimes after only a few days. Weakness is noted when the patient fails ventilator weaning. A careful search should exclude brainstem disorders (central pontine myelinolysis), acute spinal disorders, toxic myopathies, and GBS. In general, many patients have a combination of critical illness polyneuropathy (CIP) and critical weakness myopathy (CIM).

- Both CIP and CIM are associated with similar risk factors, including intubation for more than a week, prolonged neuromuscular blockade, sepsis, use of corticosteroids, and elevated blood glucose. CIP often spares the cranial nerves; deep tendon reflexes are absent, and there may be sensory loss on clinical exam. In CIP, electrophysiologic evaluation reveals an axonal motor and sensory neuropathy with low amplitudes. In CIM, NCS are normal, but myopathic units may be seen on EMG testing. CIM is the most common cause of ICU-acquired myopathy but is difficult to differentiate from CIP, as these two conditions overlap clinically, so the term ICU-acquired weakness has been used.

- There is no specific treatment known for ICU-acquired weakness. Half of the patients recover fully after a long and rigorous rehabilitation program, but the other half experience significant long-term disability.

SUGGESTED READING

Barohn RJ, Dimachkie MM, Jackson CE. A pattern recognition approach to the patient with a suspected myopathy. *Neurol Clin.* 2014;32(3):569–593.

Dhand UK. Clinical approach to the weak patient in the intensive care unit. *Respir Care.* 2006;51(9):1024–1041.

Gihus, NE. Myasthenia gravis. *N Engl J Med.* 2016;375:2570–2581.

Katirji B, Kaminski HJ, Ruff RL. *Neuromuscular Disorders in Clinical Practice.* New York, NY: Springer-Verlag; 2014.

Latronico N, Bolton CF. Critical illness polyneuropathy and myopathy: a major cause of muscle weakness and paralysis. *Lancet Neurol.* 2011;10:931–941.

Saguil A. Evaluation of the patient with muscle weakness. *Am Fam Physician.* 2005;71(7):1327–1336.

Wijdicks EFM, Klein CJ. Guillain-Barré syndrome. *Mayo Clin Proc.* 2017;92(3):467–479.

3 Subacutely Developing Weakness

Mamatha Pasnoor, Mazen M. Dimachkie, and Richard J. Barohn

HISTORY

Neuromuscular disorders refer to any condition that affects the components of the peripheral motor or sensory system, including the anterior horn cells, the muscles they innervate, the ventral root, the plexus, the peripheral nerves, and the neuromuscular junction for the motor system. Neurologic evaluation is the most important part of diagnosing a neuromuscular problem, as in any other neurologic condition. Despite vast technological advances, the history and neurologic evaluation of patients remains of foremost importance for diagnosis.

Neuromuscular diseases manifest through a combination of symptoms attributable to the dysfunction of motor or sensory nerves.

- Weakness, atrophy, muscle cramps, stiffness, fasciculations, or other abnormal muscle movements, such as myotonia, constitute the typical motor symptoms.
- Pain, paresthesias, numbness, and sensory ataxia are typical sensory symptoms.

History should focus on identifying the location, nature of the initial symptoms, and subsequent evolution of the symptoms in chronological fashion.

Muscle weakness is a common neuromuscular problem. Patients commonly use the word "weakness" in their symptom description as a synonym for asthenia. Patients with true muscle weakness usually describe the weakness in terms of the problems that result with activities of daily living. For example, patients with weakness of hip flexors will have difficulty getting in and out of the car, patients with hip abductor weakness may have waddling gait, patients with hip extensor weakness may have lordosis, patients with proximal weakness in the upper extremities may have difficulty combing their hair, and patients with distal weakness may have difficulty opening jars or buttoning shirts.

Patterns of muscle weakness and correlation with associated symptoms help with neuromuscular localization.

CLINICAL INVESTIGATION

Examination should be used to determine the presence of motor and/or sensory impairment, the pattern, and the type of involvement.

- With the motor system, deficits are identified as indicating pathology of the upper motor neuron system or lower motor neuron system or both.

- With the sensory system, if possible, characteristics that suggest preferential involvement of small or large fiber modalities should be identified.

- Recognition of the pattern and severity of muscle weakness and associated symptoms such as sensory deficits, fasciculations, and atrophy helps to determine the diagnosis.

- Testing of cranial nerve function in suspected neuromuscular disease can offer significant insight into the diagnosis. Eyelid ptosis, movements of the eyes, pupil size, and reactivity to light provide us with useful information. Neuromuscular disorders causing ophthalmoparesis that spare the pupil include neuromuscular junction disorders, diabetic third nerve palsies, and myopathic conditions. Ophthalmoparesis with pupillary involvement is seen in Guillain-Barré syndrome (GBS). Assessment of jaw, facial, and tongue strength is useful. Jaw opening weakness is usually indicative of myopathy, whereas jaw closure weakness is typical of myasthenia gravis (MG). Ventilation can also be assessed at the bedside with various techniques, with the patient either lying down or sitting up, while counting to 20 in one breath or with a spirometer.

- As with its motor counterpart, the results of the sensory examination are most credible when they are concordant with both the history and the sensory examination of small and large fiber modality. Boundaries of the sensory loss help to determine whether the condition is length dependent or non-length dependent. Sensory deficits are considered length dependent if they are present with a distal to proximal gradient of sensory loss also known as the stocking-glove pattern, whereas non-length-dependent neuropathies do not follow this pattern.

- Autonomic function testing at the bedside includes observation of pupillary responses, both to light and to nuchal stimulation; identification of dry, cracked skin, which suggests the possibility of anhidrosis; assessment of pulse variation in response to deep breathing; and most commonly, orthostatic blood pressure and pulse measurements.

Laboratory testing is ideally used to support a clinically established working diagnosis. Table 3.1 lists tests for specific conditions.

TABLE 3.1 Laboratory Testing

Laboratory evaluation of a patient with subacute weakness

Potential etiology	Tests to order
Muscle Disorders	
Myopathy due to electrolyte imbalance	CMP, CK
Rhabdomyolysis	CK, serum and urine myoglobin, CBC, CMP
Myopathy due to endocrinopathies	CK, thyroid function tests, parathyroid function tests, CMP
Inflammatory myopathies	CK, myositis specific antibodies, ESR, TSH SIFE, malignancy work up, pulmonary function tests
Necrotizing autoimmune myopathy	CK, HMGCoA reductase, myositis specific antibodies, malignancy workup
Infectious myositis	CK, CBC, CMP, Blood cultures, CXR, UA
Toxic necrotizing myopathies	Look at medication list and exposures, especially statins
Metabolic myopathies	CK, non-ischemic forearm testing, muscle biopsy with enzyme analysis, alternatively genetic testing
Neuropathies	
Neuropathy due to vitamin or mineral deficiency	Vitamin B_1, B_{12}, E, and copper
Sjögren's syndrome	SSA, SSB
Infectious neuropathy	CBC, blood cultures, HIV, FTA-Abs, TP, West Nile virus serologies, enterovirus serology CSF
Chronic immune sensory polyradiculopathy (CISP)	CSF, nerve biopsy in some cases
Mononeuritis multiplex	ESR, ANA, ANCA, hepatitis B and C serology cryoglobulins, HIV, nerve biopsy
Subacute inflammatory demyelinating neuropathy	CSF, nerve biopsy in some cases
MAG neuropathy	MAG titers
Lyme disease	Lyme serology and CSF
Hereditary neuropathy with liability to pressure palsies	PMP22 deletion
Paraproteinemia	Serum and urine immune fixation, quantitative immunoglobulins, serum free light chains, MAG antibody titers

(*continued*)

TABLE 3.1 Laboratory Testing (*continued*)

Laboratory evaluation of a patient with subacute weakness

Potential etiology	Tests to order
Lymphomatous/ carcinomatous meningitis	CSF with cytology (may need to be repeated; 3 times), muscle and nerve biopsy
Neuromuscular Junction Disorder	
Myasthenia gravis	Acetylcholine receptor (AchR) antibodies, muscle-specific tyrosine kinase antibodies, LRP4
Lambert-Eaton myasthenic syndrome	P/Q type Voltage-gated calcium-channel antibodies (VGCC)
Others	
Primary systemic amyloidosis	Serum immunofixation electrophoresis, quantitative immunoglobulin, serum free light chain assay Tissue biopsy: skin, fat, rectal, or other affected organ
Sarcoid	Serum ACE, CSF, imaging
Autonomic ganglionopathy	Acetylcholine receptor ganglionic neuronal antibodies, voltage-gated potassium autoantibodies, GAD-65 antibodies, anti-Hu antibodies
Negative results but rapidly progressive disease or severe disabling motor or sensory large fiber disease	Muscle and nerve biopsy

ACE, angiotensin-converting enzyme; ANA, antinuclear Ab; ANCA, antineu-trophilic cytoplasmic Ab; CBC, complete blood count; CK, creatine kinase; CMP, complete metabolic profile, CSF, cerebrospinal fluid; CXR, chest x-ray; ESR, erythrocyte sedimentation rate; FTA-Abs, fluorescent treponemal anti-body absorption; HMGCoA, 3-hydroxy-3-methylglutaryl-coenzyme A; LRP4, lipoprotein receptor–related protein 4; MAG, myelin-associated glycoprotein; PMP22, peripheral myelin protein 22; SIFE, serum immunofixation electrophore-sis; TP, triphosphatase; TSH, thyroid stimulating hormone, UA, urinalysis.

- Total blood count and complete metabolic profile (CMP) are useful for all conditions.
- Genetic testing is available for most of the hereditary conditions. DNA mutational analysis and biochemical testing for inborn errors of metabolism are used in specific disease conditions.

In addition to the labs, imaging may be necessary for diagnostic purposes in a few of these conditions.

- Computed tomography (CT) of the chest is required in MG to look for thymoma. CT of the chest, abdomen, and pelvis may be necessary for malignancy workup in polymyositis, necrotizing myopathy and dermatomyositis.

- Magnetic resonance imaging (MRI) is useful to assess mononeuropathies, radiculopathies, and plexopathies and can also be used in myositis to identify inflammation and determine the muscle to biopsy.
- Neuromuscular ultrasonography is a quicker and more dynamic imaging method to test for entrapment neuropathies—and for muscle disorders. Magnetic resonance neurography is increasingly being used for peripheral nerve disease.

Other tests useful for neuromuscular diagnosis include electromyography (EMG) and nerve conduction studies (NCS), collectively known as electrodiagnostic (EDX) testing; quantitative sensory testing (QST); autonomic nervous system testing (ANST); and muscle and nerve biopsies. These tests are discussed in detail elsewhere in this text.

DIFFERENTIAL DIAGNOSIS

Many neuromuscular disorders present with acute/subacute presentations (Table 3.2). The approach to neuromuscular disorders, as with any other neurologic condition, should include determining the site of the lesion, the cause of the lesion (Figure 3.1), and initiating specific therapy. In the absence of specific therapy, it is important to initiate supportive care and management.

The examiner can localize the neuromuscular weakness to one of the following four sites:

1. Neuronopathy (involving the cell bodies) which can be either motor, sensory, or autonomic
2. Neuropathy with involvement of either the root, plexus, or peripheral nerve
3. Neuromuscular junction disorder
4. Myopathy
   - Sensory nerve involvement is usually suspected if the patient has sensory symptoms (tingling, numbness, or pain). Motor nerve involvement causes weakness that can be either symmetric or asymmetric.
   - Motor neuron cell body (neuronopathy) involvement causes asymmetric weakness, asymmetric atrophy, fasciculations, or cramps.
   - Muscle or neuromuscular junction involvement is suspected if the patient presents with proximal weakness, sometime hypertrophy of the muscles, or ocular involvement (orbicularis oculi weakness, ptosis, ocular motility). Patients with neuromuscular junction disorders also present with fluctuations in their symptoms.

TABLE 3.2 Neuromuscular Disorders Presenting With Subacute Weakness

Anterior horn cell
Poliomyelitis
Peripheral neuropathy
Subacute inflammatory demyelinating polyneuropathy
Porphyria
Diphtheria
Tick paralysis
Toxic neuropathies
Diabetic amyotrophy
Vasculitis
Carcinomatous infiltration (e.g., leukemia and lymphoma)
Paraneoplastic neuropathy
Neuromuscular junction
Botulism
Lambert-Eaton myasthenic syndrome
Myasthenia gravis
Myopathy
Periodic paralysis
Electrolyte imbalance
Endocrinopathies
Inflammatory myopathies
Dermatomyositis
Polymyositis
Infectious myositis
Toxic myopathies
Metabolic myopathies
Glycogen and lipid disorders

Based on the history and examination of a patient presenting with subacute weakness, it is important to determine:

1. The systems involved: motor, sensory, autonomic, or a combination thereof.

   - If the patient has weakness without sensory loss, a motor neuronopathy or motor neuron disease is most likely. The differential diagnosis for patients presenting with an acute/subacute onset

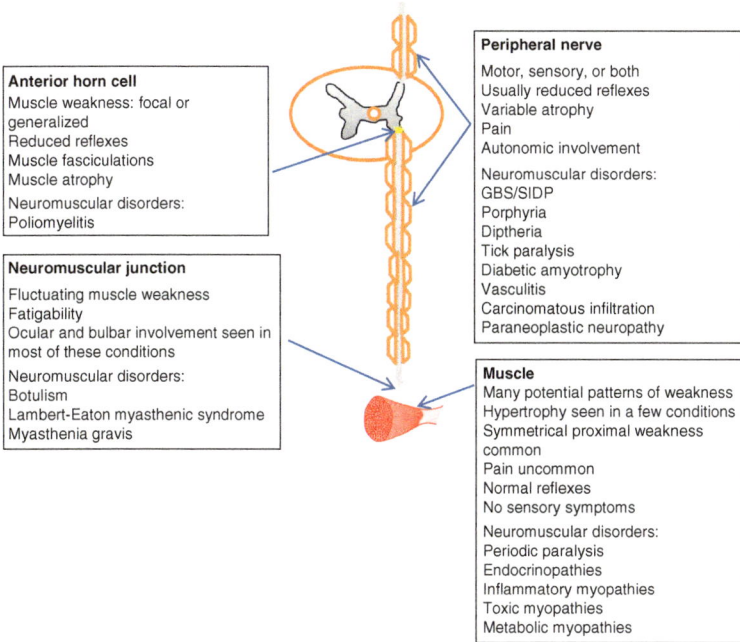

FIGURE 3.1 Presentation of neuromuscular conditions based on localization.

Peripheral nerve

Motor, sensory, or both
Usually reduced reflexes
Variable atrophy
Pain
Autonomic involvement

Neuromuscular disorders:
GBS/SIDP
Porphyria
Diptheria
Tick paralysis
Diabetic amyotrophy
Vasculitis
Carcinomatous infiltration
Paraneoplastic neuropathy

Anterior horn cell

Muscle weakness: focal or generalized
Reduced reflexes
Muscle fasciculations
Muscle atrophy

Neuromuscular disorders:
Poliomyelitis

Neuromuscular junction

Fluctuating muscle weakness
Fatigability
Ocular and bulbar involvement seen in most of these conditions

Neuromuscular disorders:
Botulism
Lambert-Eaton myasthenic syndrome
Myasthenia gravis

Muscle

Many potential patterns of weakness
Hypertrophy seen in a few conditions
Symmetrical proximal weakness common
Pain uncommon
Normal reflexes
No sensory symptoms

Neuromuscular disorders:
Periodic paralysis
Endocrinopathies
Inflammatory myopathies
Toxic myopathies
Metabolic myopathies

includes poliomyelitis, GBS, subacute demyelinating polyradic-uloneuropathy (SIDP), lead intoxication, and acute porphyria.

- If the patient has chronic sensory loss without motor involvement, consider hereditary sensory neuropathy or early signs of any neuropathy but acutely consider the Miller Fisher syndrome.
- If the patient has autonomic symptoms, consider diabetes mellitus, amyloidosis, GBS or its variants, and idiopathic or autoimmune pandysautonomia. Hereditary sensory autonomic neuropathy and hereditary autonomic neuropathy have a chronic presentation.

2. The distribution of weakness: distal versus distal and proximal, focal asymmetric versus symmetric, and focal midline versus proximal symmetric (neck/trunk/bulbar/diaphragm) involvement. With distal weakness, patients usually report tripping, being unable to hold objects, or dropping objects held in the hand. Patients with proximal weakness report difficulty getting up from a chair and difficulty raising their arms for brushing their teeth or combing their hair.

- Distal symmetric weakness with sensory symptoms is seen with axonal peripheral neuropathy, which is most likely to be due to metabolic conditions and less likely to be treatable.

However, variants of acquired demyelinating neuropathies can present in this manner.

- Distal symmetric weakness without sensory symptoms (purely motor) usually occurs in chronic conditions such as muscular dystrophies, myopathies, and hereditary motor neuropathies. Some patients with hereditary neuropathy do not have sensory symptoms even though we can see sensory loss on examination. MG can sometimes present with distal weakness only, especially finger extension.

- Distal and proximal symmetric weakness with sensory symptoms is usually seen with acquired immune demyelinating polyneuropathies. These usually respond to immunosuppression or immunomodulation.

- Distal and proximal weakness that is symmetric without sensory symptoms is seen in spinal muscular atrophy, some myopathies, and limb-girdle muscular dystrophies. Most of these conditions are chronic.

- Asymmetric weakness without sensory symptoms is seen with motor neuron disease.

- Asymmetric weakness with sensory symptoms is seen with lumbosacral or cervical radiculoplexopathies, vasculitis, radiculopathies, plexopathies, compressive mononeuropathies, and leprosy.

- Focal weakness, such as neck extensor weakness, as well as bulbar weakness can be seen with motor neuron diseases, neuromuscular junction disorders (MG, Lambert-Eaton myasthenic syndrome), and some myopathies such as isolated neck extensor muscles (INEMs).

3. Sensory symptoms: numbness, tingling, severe pain, severe proprioceptive loss (asymmetric without weakness or symmetric), sensory loss without sensory symptoms.

- Subacute-onset neuropathies associated with distal pain include neuropathy due to diabetes mellitus, vasculitis, subacute acquired demyelinating neuropathy, amyloidosis, toxic neuropathies (arsenic, thallium), HIV-related polyneuropathy, and Fabry's disease.

- Sensory (and motor) symptoms associated with back pain are seen with radiculoplexopathies (diabetic amyotrophy), radiculopathies, acquired demyelinating polyneuropathies, and carcinomatous infiltration of the roots.

- Severe proprioceptive loss and vibratory loss with resulting balance problems and normal strength are seen with sensory neuronopathy also known as ganglionopathy. Causes of sensory ganglionopathies include cancer (paraneoplastic such as anti-Hu syndrome), Sjögren syndrome, idiopathic sensory neuronopathy, treatment with cis-platinum and other analogues, vitamin B_6 toxicity, HIV-related sensory neuronopathy, and posterior column damage due to subacute combined degeneration. Sensory nerve and dorsal column involvement is seen in vitamin E deficiency.

- Brisk reflexes and sensory symptoms can be seen with involvement of the peripheral sensory nerves and spinal cord. This is commonly encountered with myeloneuropathy due to vitamin B_{12} deficiency and copper deficiency.
- Loss of pain, light touch, and temperature sensations is seen with small fiber neuropathies, hereditary sensory neuropathy, Fabry's disease, and some cases of amyloidosis.

4. The temporal evolution: acute (days to 4 weeks), subacute (4 to 8 weeks), chronic (greater than 8 weeks), any preceding events, drugs.

- Acute and subacute presentations are seen with acquired inflammatory demyelinating neuropathy, vasculitis, and diabetic amyotrophy (Table 3.2). A relapsing course can be seen with porphyria.
- Chronic conditions are discussed in a separate chapter.

5. Evidence on the physical examination suggesting a hereditary neuropathy—for example, hammertoes and pes cavus, abnormal examination findings in family members. These are mostly chronic conditions and are discussed in other chapters.

6. Evidence on the physical exam of upper motor neuron involvement, either with or without sensory loss. Upper motor involvement is manifested by examination findings of brisk reflexes, Babinski sign or Hoffman reflex.

- Asymmetric upper motor involvement without sensory loss is seen with motor neuron disease (amyotrophic lateral sclerosis).
- Symmetric upper motor involvement with sensory loss is seen with myeloneuropathy associated with vitamin B_{12} deficiency and copper deficiency.

Pattern Recognition

The key to diagnosis of neuromuscular conditions is recognition of a clinical pattern. Barohn and Amato described 10 different patterns of neuropathic disorders.

1. Symmetric proximal and distal weakness with sensory loss is suggestive of acquired demyelinating neuropathy. Consider GBS with acute onset, subacute inflammatory demyelinating polyneuropathy (SIDP), and chronic inflammatory demyelinating polyneuropathy (CIDP).

- Subacute inflammatory demyelinating polyneuropathy: GBS or acute inflammatory demyelinating polyneuropathy (AIDP) and chronic CIDP are discussed in other chapters. Progression of symptoms beyond 4 weeks up to 8 weeks is considered SIDP.

According to Oh et al. (1), for a diagnosis of "definite SIDP," there were four mandatory criteria: (a) progressive motor and/or sensory dysfunction consistent with neuropathy in more than one limb, with time to nadir between 4 and 8 weeks; (b) electrophysiological evidence of demyelination in at least two nerves; (c) no other etiology of neuropathy; and (d) no relapse on adequate follow-up. Supportive criteria include high spinal fluid protein level (more than 55 mg/dL) and inflammatory cells in the nerve biopsy. A diagnosis of "probable SIDP" requires progression of demyelinating neuropathy over a 4- to 8-week period. The two most common presentations of SIDP are symmetric motor-sensory neuropathy and pure motor neuropathy. Cranial nerve involvement and respiratory failure are rare. According to the literature, definite SIDP has all the characteristics of CIDP with three exceptions: a higher rate of antecedent infection, no relapse rate, and a high rate of recovery to normal. Most of these patients, unlike patients with GBS, may require prednisone and other immunotherapies for their management.

2. Symmetric distal sensory loss with or without weakness. Consider these conditions.
   - Metabolic disorders such as distal symmetric polyneuropathy due to impaired glucose tolerance and diabetes mellitus
     - Diabetic neuropathy is the most common type of neuropathy. The common presentation is distal symmetric polyneuropathy with "glove" and "stocking" distribution of sensory loss, decreased vibratory sensation, and decreased or normal proprioception at the toes. Weakness of the feet and toes is rare and usually seen with severe neuropathy. Various presentations are seen with diabetic neuropathy, including mononeuropathies, asymmetric lumbosacral radiculoplexopathies, radiculopathies, and autonomic neuropathies that can present with subacute onset. The distal symmetric polyneuropathy has a slow chronic progressive course. Metabolic, vascular, inflammatory, and immune theories have been suggested for its pathogenesis. Axonal and demyelinating patterns of sensorimotor involvement can be seen on electrophysiology. Treatment is mainly aimed at glycemic control and neuropathic pain management.
   - Drugs and toxins
     - Toxic neuropathy caused by drug ingestion, drug or chemical abuse, or industrial chemical exposure from the workplace or the environment. Distal axonopathy, causing dying-back axonal degeneration, is the most common form. Some of the substances that cause subacute-onset neuropathy include arsenic, hexacarbons, lead, mercury, thalium, and metronidazole.

o Arsenic exposure can be due to environmental exposure such as mining, exposure to by-products of copper, and lead smelting. Ingestion of trivalent arsenic can be as a result of suicidal ideation, homicide, food, or water contamination. In addition, Chinese herbal preparations and certain marine organisms may contain large amounts of arsenic. Patients usually have a garlic-like odor to their breath and tissue fluids, vomiting, diarrhea, tachycardia, and hypotension secondary to fluid loss. Massive overdose usually causes subacute neuropathy. Onset of neuropathy is usually 10 to 20 days after exposure. Patients develop distal paresthesias and numbness that progress over 2 to 5 weeks; sensory symptoms are more prominent than motor symptoms. Diagnosis is based on arsenic levels in urine. Arsenic deposits can also be found in other tissues, such has hair and fingernails, with chronic exposure. EDX testing and pathology show distal axonal loss with or without some demyelination. Chelation with BAL or penicillamine for few months is the treatment with slow recovery over years.

o Hexacarbons: *n*-Hexane, *n*-butyl ketone is converted to 2,5-hexanedione, which is the active agent. Exposure is seen with glue-sniffing, gasoline-sniffing, and occupational exposure. The exposure route is usually airborne, but occasionally through the skin. Hexacarbon exposure is commonly seen in young males, and some occupational exposure–related toxicity is seen in auto mechanics, printing plants, sandal shops, and furniture factories. Exposure leads to subacute or slow progressive neuropathy that develops over 2 months. Patients have distal sensory loss, some distal (more than proximal) weakness in the legs, and symmetric, absent or preserved reflexes. They have a delayed recording after removal of the toxin. Progression occurs over 1 to 4 months, and takes months to years to improve. Other symptoms include encephalopathy, weight loss, malaise, anorexia, and abdominal pain. EDX testing shows axonal loss with some features of demyelination. Nerve biopsy may be normal or show giant neuro-filamentous swellings. Treatment is removal of the exposure.

o Lead: Lead toxicity is common in children, especially those who live in homes built from 1920 to 1950. Industrial exposure is also a source of toxicity. Exposure occurs with ingestion and inhalation. Ingestion of moonshine, whiskey, rum, products processed in lead pipes, and some Asian folk medicines can cause toxicity. Occupational exposure is seen with smelting, battery manufacture, demolition, auto radiator, and silver refining. Toxic levels are defined in children as greater than 10 µg/dL, and in adults as greater than 30 µg/dL. Distal (more than proximal) asymmetric weakness is seen. Severe exposure may cause quadriplegia. Focal weakness may affect the wrist and finger extensors, proximal shoulder, hand intrinsic, peroneal, and laryngeal muscles. Abdominal pain, fatigue, irritability, and anemia are seen. Lethargy, ataxia, dysarthria, renal failure, hypertension, and seizures can be seen. Chronic low-level exposure leads to distal sensory involvement. Diagnosis is based on blue discoloration of the gums, mild anemia, basophilic stippling of erythrocytes, and high urine coproporphyrin levels (greater than 0.2 mg/L). Symptoms are usually seen at blood levels of greater than 80 µg/dL. Radiographic evidence includes lead lines on bones. Motor axonal loss with mild slowing of conduction velocities is seen on EDX testing. Pathology shows axonal degeneration, segmental demyelination, and endoneurial edema. Slow improvement occurs with treatment. Treatment involves elimination of exposure and administration of penicillamine, succimer, CaNa$_2$ EDT, BAL, or Dimerval.

○ Mercury: Exposure can be airborne or through gastrointestinal absorption. Patients develop encephalopathy, peripheral nerve toxicity, early paresthesias, and ataxia. Exposure to metallic mercury vapor causes motor axonal neuropathy and myokymia. Other effects of mercury exposure include increased excitability, postural tremor, mouth inflammation, fetid breath, erosive bronchitis, interstitial pneumonitis, pulmonary edema, renal insufficiency, psychosis, extrapyramidal signs, ataxia, and postural tremor. Sensory more than motor involvement, and distal leg more than arm involvement are seen. Patients have pain and paresthesias, absent tendon reflexes at the ankles, and distal weakness in the feet. EDX testing reveals small-amplitude SNAPs and chronic denervation findings on needle EMG. Diagnosis is made by examining the 24-hour urinary excretion. Treatment is with chelation therapy and spironolactone.

○ Thallium: Used in rodenticides and insecticides. Toxicity is due to homicide and accidental ingestion. Onset of neuropathy is usually greater than 1 week after exposure. Patients usually develop vomiting, diarrhea, and abdominal pain, followed by burning paresthesias in the legs and joint pain. Mild distal weakness may be seen, but tendon reflexes may be preserved. Hair loss occurs after 2 to 6 weeks. Coma, lethargy, and cardiac and respiratory failure may occur with acute exposure. Tachycardia, hypertension, scalp alopecia, and hyperkeratosis are other signs and symptoms. Pathology shows distal axonopathy and swollen mitochondria. Diagnosis is based on urine and tissue thallium. Recovery occurs over 6 months. Treatment involves administration of potassium chloride or Prussian blue.

- o Metronidazole: This antibiotic and antiprotozoal agent is used for inflammatory bowel disease. Chronic drug usage for months to years, especially with a total dose greater than 30 grams, leads to development of neuropathy, which can be subacute or chronic sensory neuropathy. Distal symmetric sensory neuropathy with pain and burning may be seen. Other associated findings include cardiomyopathy, taste abnormality, neutropenia, and thrombocytopenia. EDX testing reveals axonal sensory and motor neuropathy. Sympathetic skin response may be reduced or absent. Protein level in the cerebrospinal fluid (CSF) may be high. Pathology shows axonal loss of large myelinated fibers. Complete or partial recovery is seen 6 to 12 months after stopping the drug. In some patients, neuropathy may progress even after stopping the drug, which is known as coasting phenomenon.

- Sjögren's neuropathy: This autoimmune condition, which is seen in adults, causes dry eyes and dry mouth. Sensory non-length-dependent neuropathy is the most common presentation of Sjögren neuropathy, which is usually managed with neuropathic medications. However, some people may develop mononeuritis multiplex, a more severe neuropathy with significant weakness and pain with very abrupt onset of weakness. Skin biopsy is used to diagnose small fiber neuropathy in these patients. Immunosuppressive medications are used for mononeuritis multiplex presentation.

- Sarcoid neuropathy: Prevalence of sarcoidosis is about 1 to 40 cases per 100,000 persons, and this disease is 10 times more common in the African American population. The age of onset is usually around 20 to 40 years. Erythema nodosum is seen on the skin; ocular symptoms, interstitial lung disease, arthritis, thoracic lymphadenopathy, hypercalcemia, and lacrimal gland enlargement are other features of sarcoidosis. Genetic associations have been described. Familial risk is increased 5-fold in siblings and 18-fold in White siblings, but is lower in African American siblings. About 10% of patients develop neuropathy, with this outcome being more common in White females. The mean age of onset is around 46 years. Patients develop paresthesias and sensory loss that can be non-length dependent, involving the face, trunk, and limbs. There is mostly small-fiber involvement. Patients have pain, burning sensations, and intermittent numbness. Few patients develop weakness more in the legs than in the arms. Tendon reflexes are reduced at the ankles. Autonomic features are seen in about 50% of the patients. Cranial nerve involvement is uncommon and usually demonstrates slow progression. EDX study shows axonal loss, and the Quantitative Sudomotor Axon Reflex Test (QSART) can be abnormal in some patients. Nerve pathology shows granulomas and axonal loss. Skin biopsy shows reduced fiber density. Treatment is intravenous immunoglobulin (IVIG) and anti-tumor necrosis factor (anti-TNF) drugs.

- Sarcoidosis can mimic the presentation of GBS, vasculitic neuropathy, and radiculopathies.
- Hereditary neuropathies: Amyloid, hereditary sensory neuropathy (HSN, Fabry's disease, Nav 1.7, Charcot-Marie-Tooth [CMT] disease) causes chronic neuropathies and is discussed in another chapter.
- Vasculitis: Vasculitic neuropathy is a rare cause of neuropathy but an important cause of axonal neuropathy due to its potential treatment implications. A peripheral neuropathy task force classified the vasculitides associated with neuropathy into three groups: primary systemic, secondary systemic, and nonsystemic cause. Vasculitis is common in males older than age 50 years and has an acute to subacute presentation. Several anatomic patterns of neuropathy have been described:
  - Mononeuritis multiplex, in which individual nerves are affected, most commonly the peroneal nerves (90%). The posterior tibial, ulnar, median, and radial nerves are also affected.
  - Confluent mononeuritis multiplex, which is characterized by distal asymmetric, motor, and sensory loss.
  - Distal symmetric pattern.

Patients present with severe pain and burning dysesthesias with weakness of muscles in that nerve distribution. Fever, weight loss, arthralgias, and fatigue are commonly seen with systemic vasculitis. EDX testing reveals multifocal changes, axonal loss, and conduction block in the acute phase. Biopsy of nerve and muscle shows epineurial inflammation, necrosis of the vessel wall with inflammatory cells, luminal narrowing, vessel recanalization, and focal calcification of walls with an increased number of epineurial vessels. Patchy involvement with differential fascicular loss of axons is also seen. Prognosis is good overall with nonsystemic vasculitic neuropathy. Treatment includes prednisone, solumedrol, cyclophosphamide, methotrexate, and management of systemic vasculitis.

3. Asymmetric distal weakness with sensory loss. This can occur with single nerve or multiple nerve involvement.

- Single nerve: Compressive neuropathy: Clinical history and examination findings are usually sufficient to establish the diagnosis of compressive or entrapment neuropathy. Compression of the peripheral nerves results in pain, paresthesias, and loss of function of that nerve. Compression may occur in any peripheral nerve, but considerations such as anatomic course, superficial location, and adjacent fibrous or osseous structures may increase the predisposition to compression injury. Mechanical pressure leads to ischemia and associated edema of the compressed nerve. Acute compression leads to focal demyelination and Wallerian-like axonal degeneration. In cases of acute or subacute compression-related neuropathies such as Saturday night palsy (radial neuropathy at the spiral groove), treatment is usually supportive and improvement is expected over time without any intervention. Coexistent systemic medical conditions—for example, diabetes and thyroid diseases—may predispose an individual to development of entrapment neuropathy. EDX testing is helpful in confirming the diagnosis, determining the severity, and excluding mimicking conditions. Peripheral nerve imaging technologies, including ultrasonography and magnetic resonance imaging, may provide additional information, particularly in atypical cases. Conservative management is usually effective, but sometimes surgical release is necessary.

- Radiculopathy: Caused by compression or irritation of the nerve as it exits the spinal column. Symptoms include pain, numbness, tingling, and weakness in the arms and legs. Patients respond well to conservative management including medications, physical therapy, or chiropractic treatment. Radiculopathy can resolve within 6 weeks to 3 months. Some patients need surgical management.

- Multiple nerves: mononeuritis multiplex, vasculitis, hereditary neuropathy with pressure palsies (HNPP) infectious (Lyme disease, leprosy, HIV, sarcoidosis, hepatitis), and multifocal motor neuropathy (MMN). Multifocal acquired demyelinating sensory and motor (MADSAM) neuropathy, also known as Lewis-Sumner syndrome, presents as a chronic condition.

- Mononeuritis multiplex can be seen in various conditions, including diabetes mellitus, vasculitis, amyloidosis, direct tumor involvement, infections, drug hypersensitivity, and paraneoplastic syndromes.

4. Asymmetric proximal and distal weakness with sensory loss: polyradiculopathy, plexopathy, radiculoplexopathy.

- Parsonage-Turner syndrome, also known as brachial neuritis or neuralgic amyotrophy, is a peripheral nerve disorder that causes severe pain, usually involving the shoulder and the arm. The pain is followed in days to weeks by weakness. The muscles most commonly involved are the upper trunk and brachial plexus muscles, but any nerve in the arm or even the leg can be involved. This syndrome can develop after viral illness, immunization, mild trauma, physical exertion, or surgery, but often the cause is not obvious. The most common theory as to its cause is that it is a viral-induced, immune-mediated process. EDX testing shows evidence of upper trunk brachial plexopathy. The vast majority of patients with Parsonage-Turner syndrome recover without any treatment. Strength and pain improve. In patients who do not recover, a surgical option may be considered about 6 to 9 months later.

- Diabetic lumbosacral radiculoplexus neuropathy, also known as diabetic amyotrophy, is a proximal diabetic neuropathy. It is rare and has a subacute presentation. It occurs in patients with poorly controlled diabetes mellitus. Patients present with severe pain in the back and proximally in the thigh at the onset, followed by proximal weakness, especially quadriceps and psoas weakness. Sensory loss is not prominent. The symptoms continue for few months and then either plateau or improve spontaneously even without any treatment.

5. Asymmetric distal weakness without sensory loss that has a subacute onset of symptoms.

   - With upper motor neuron findings: amyotrophic lateral sclerosis

   - Without upper motor neuron findings: MMN, poliomyelitis, polio-like conditions (e.g., West Nile virus, enterovirus 68)

     ▪ Amyotrophic lateral sclerosis (ALS): This includes hereditary and sporadic forms. Prevalence is about 3 to 8 cases per 100,000 people. Risk increases with age up to 74 years. ALS is more common in males than in females. Many factors have been associated with increased risk of ALS, including head trauma, smoking, diabetes, military service, and varsity athletics; however, no definite etiology has been identified. A number of genes have been associated with ALS. Detailed information on each gene is beyond the scope of this chapter. Patients usually present with asymmetric-onset limb weakness with muscle loss, muscle twitches, and muscle cramps, with or without bulbar symptoms. Some patients present with a bulbar onset with dysarthria, dysphagia, jaw weakness, tongue atrophy, and fasciculations. Others present with respiratory failure at the onset or with progression of the condition. Examination findings include dysarthria and weakness of the tongue, facial muscles, neck, and extremities. Atrophy and fasciculations are seen in the affected muscles. Brisk reflexes are usually present, although with severe weakness of the muscles, the reflexes may become difficult to assess in the extremities. Jaw reflex is also brisk in these patients. Plantar response is extensor. Inappropriate laughter or crying due to pseudobulbar affect is seen in these individuals. Fronto-temporal dementia occurs in 3% to 15% of patients. Median survival in ALS is 36 months. Diagnosis is usually made clinically, and EMG/NCS is used to provide supportive evidence of lower motor neuron involvement. NCS show low amplitude of motor responses; EMG shows diffuse and widespread denervation and reinnervation changes with fasciculation potentials. Sensory responses are normal. The cause of death is usually respiratory failure. Treatment is mainly symptomatic. Riluzole may increase survival by an average of 3 months.

- Poliomyelitis: This infection is caused by an enterovirus, a member of a subgroup of picornaviridae, that afflicts children and adults, particularly those living in third world countries. The virus is transmitted through the fecal–oral route and spreads from the lymphatics to the blood and then to the CNS. The virus replicates and releases RNA into the cytoplasm. Polio outbreaks are most common in late summer, and usually affect children between 6 months to 3 years of age. About 90% to 95% of patients are asymptomatic with viremia after viral exposure, but minor illness with fever, malaise, and sore throat occurs 1 to 5 days after exposure, and major illness with aseptic meningitis, fever, headache, stiff neck, and back pain occurs 4 to 20 days postinfection. Paralytic disease occurs in 50% of patients with major illness (0.1%–1% of infected patients). Acute or subacute onset of focal or asymmetric proximal weakness, more in the legs than in the arms, and bulbar involvement are observed. Examination reveals brisk reflexes in early cases, with these reflexes being reduced in the affected limbs after 12 to 20 hours. Muscle atrophy can be seen after 2 to 3 weeks. Maximal improvement occurs in 6 to 9 months. Residual weakness is seen in 60% to 70% of patients. Autonomic symptoms, pain, and fasciculations may be seen. Mortality in children is 2% to 5%; in adults, it is 15% to 30%. CSF analysis reveals acutely polymorphonuclear pleocytosis and increased protein. EDX testing shows decreased motor amplitudes and increased spontaneous activity. Pathology shows perivascular inflammation, loss of anterior horn cells, abnormal morphology, and chromatolysis. Chronically, and a few decades after the acute illness, progressive weakness in the most affected limbs of polio survivors is indicative of postpolio muscular atrophy. This later manifests on EMG as giant motor unit potentials in addition to active denervation.

- West Nile virus and enterovirus infections have a similar presentation to poliomyelitis and are more likely to be seen in the present day than poliomyelitis. Besides Dengue, another emerging neurotrophic virus is the Zika virus, which can present as either GBS or as an acute infectious painful neuritis.

6. Symmetric sensory loss (with or without distal weakness) and upper motor neuron signs.

- Myeloneuropathy: Vitamin B_{12} deficiency, copper deficiency, end stage liver disease
   - Myeloneuropathy: This disease process affects both the spinal cord and the peripheral nerves. The causes include autoimmune disorders, tumors, toxins, and vitamin deficiencies. Vitamin B_{12} deficiency is the most classic form of myeloneuropathy due to nutritional deficiency. Vitamin B_{12} deficiency sometimes occurs in long-standing vegetarians or vegans due to decreased intake. More commonly, it occurs due to poor absorption in the small intestine. In some people, this condition may be due to autoimmune disease in which antibodies attack the cells that secrete intrinsic factor. Decreased absorption due to gastrointestinal (GI) surgeries or GI diseases can lead to deficiency. Some medications, such as metformin, also can lower vitamin B_{12} levels. Myelopathy caused by low vitaimin B_{12} is also called subacute combined degeneration. Posterior columns in the spinal cord are involved. Autonomic nervous symptoms involvement may be seen. Distal symmetric peripheral neuropathy is seen. Dementia can occur with severe long-standing deficiency. Deficiency can be confirmed by measuring the vitamin level. EDX testing shows axonal sensorimotor polyneuropathy. Magnetic resonance imaging, somatosensory evoked potentials, and visual-evoked potentials may show abnormalities. Oral or intramuscular vitamin B_{12} injections are used to treat the condition. Typically, it requires lifelong supplementation with vitamin B_{12}. Copper deficiency presents with myeloneuropathy similar to that seen with vitamin B_{12} deficiency.

7. Symmetric weakness without sensory loss

- Subacute onset is seen in myopathies and neuromuscular junction disorders.
   - Neuromuscular junction disorders
      o Myasthenia gravis: This autoimmune condition affects the neuromuscular junction. A chronic condition, MG is associated with intermittent acute/subacute worsening, reported as exacerbation. Patients present with fluctuating

weakness in the extremities, or with bulbar, ocular, or generalized weakness. Two peaks are seen in adult MG: (a) early, in the second to fifth decades of life; and (b) late, in the sixth to ninth decades. The early peak has female predominance, whereas late disease is seen in more males with increasing age. Prevalence is 77.7 cases per million. Patients present with fluctuating weakness, which can be ocular, bulbar, confined to the extremities, or generalized. Examination findings may include ptosis, diplopia with restricted extraocular movements, weakness of the facial muscles, jaw weakness, dysarthria, and weakness of the extremity muscles, with normal sensory examination and normal reflexes. Shortness of breath may be present in some people. The hallmark of this condition is the increase in weakness seen with activity. Diagnostic tests include testing for acetylcholine receptor antibodies in the blood, muscle-specific tyrosine kinase (MuSK) antibodies, and recently discovered LRP4 antibodies. Edrophonium testing can be performed at the bedside if the patient has significant ptosis. The ice pack test is used by many ophthalmologists. Acetylcholinesterase is inhibited in cold temperatures, thereby increasing the availability of acetylcholine in the neuromuscular junction. Repetitive nerve stimulation and single fiber EMG (SFEMG) are also performed for diagnosis. Chest CT is performed to look for thymoma. Pulmonary function testing should be performed to assess the respiratory function. Forced vital capacity and negative inspiratory force are checked frequently and evaluate respectively the intercostal muscles and the diaphragm. Several medications are available to control MG, including anticholinesterase agents such as pyridostigmine, immunosuppressive drugs such as prednisone, azathioprine, cyclosporine, mycophenolate mofetil, tacrolimus, IV immunoglobulin, plasma exchange, and rituximab. None, except for Mestinon, are FDA-approved for MG.

8. Focal midline proximal symmetric weakness
   - Neck or trunk extensor weakness: ALS, overlap pattern: MG, INEM weakness, isolated thoracic extensor muscle weakness (ITEM)
   - Bulbar weakness: ALS/primary lateral sclerosis (PLS), isolated bulbar ALS (IBALS), Kennedy's syndrome; X-linked, bulbospinal spinal muscular atrophy (SMA), bulbar-onset GBS, overlap pattern (MG, OPD)
   - Diaphragm weakness: ALS, overlap pattern, MG, Pompe disease
     - INEM: Also known as dropped head syndrome, this nonprogressive myopathy is characterized by severe neck extensor

weakness. This relatively benign condition may be confused with more ominous neuromuscular disorders that also present with prominent neck weakness—for example, MG, ALS. INEM is characterized by severe weakness of the neck extensors, with milder weakness of the shoulder girdle and proximal arm muscles. EMG shows low-amplitude motor unit potentials in the cervical paraspinal muscles. Laboratory testing is usually unremarkable. Muscle biopsy of the cervical paraspinal muscles may show nonspecific myopathic features without inflammation. Weakness does not respond to prednisone. This condition usually has a benign course, with initial progression over few months and then stabilization in 3 to 5 months.

9. Asymmetric proprioceptive loss without weakness

Consider sensory neuronopathy due to cancer (paraneoplastic), Sjögren syndrome, vitamin B_6 toxicity, cis-platinum, HIV-related, idiopathic, vitamin E deficiency (probably nerve, not cell body).

10. Autonomic dysfunction (e.g., orthostasis, impotence, abnormal gastric motility and sweating)

DM, amyloidosis, GBS, acute autonomic ganglionopathy, Sjögren syndrome, Fabry's, porphyria, HIV-related autonomic neuropathy, idiopathic pandysautonomia (Nav 1.7 mutation), paraneoplastic.

- Acute pandysautonomia is characterized by the acute or subacute development of severe sympathetic and parasympathetic autonomic dysfunction, with preservation of somatic motor and sensory functions. A prodrome of febrile or viral illness may precede the onset of illness. The symptoms evolve over a period of a few days or weeks, but may be more gradual. Initial nonspecific symptoms of lethargy, fatigue, headache, and decreased initiative are followed by orthostatic light-headedness, blurring of vision, abdominal pain, diarrhea, dryness of eyes, and disturbed micturition. Syncope, blurred near-vision, urinary retention or incontinence, abdominal colic, distention, and at times ileus are the most disabling symptoms. Other variants have been recognized— for example, cholinergic dysautonomia, acute autonomic and sensory neuropathy. Etiology is unknown, but several factors favor an immune etiology (antecedent viral infection, elevated CSF protein). Recent studies have demonstrated the presence of antibodies to ganglionic nicotinic acetylcholine receptors (nAChR) in patients with subacute idiopathic and paraneoplastic autonomic neuropathies. Autonomic function tests are useful to confirm this condition. The disease is self-limiting, and partial or complete recovery occurs slowly over several months to years. The treatment is mainly symptomatic and supportive until spontaneous recovery occurs.

11. Cranial nerve involvement (usually 3, 4, 5, 6, or 7)
    - Isolated benign (idiopathic, diabetes)
    - Multiple—cancer, infection, sarcoid, or autoimmune
      - Immune: acute: GBS; chronic: cranial nerves 5, 7, and some-times 12; facial-onset sensory and motor neuronopathy
12. Cramps and fasciculations: mostly benign, rare cases with voltage-gated K^+ antibodies

Myopathy: Based on the history and examination, determine:
- Whether patients have negative (weakness, fatigue, atrophy) or positive (pain, cramps, contractures, stiffness/inability to relax, rippling/mounding, hypertrophy) symptoms.
- Onset and progression: acute versus subacute versus chronic, constant or episodic, monophasic or relapsing, age at onset, lifelong (congenital), progressive or nonprogressive.
- Distribution of the weakness and stiffness if present
  - Proximal
  - Distal arms/legs
  - Proximal and distal
  - Neck
  - Cranial
    - o Ocular—ptosis, extraocular muscle motility
    - o Pharyngeal—dysarthria/dysphagia
    - o Facial
  - Atrophy/hypertrophy
- Triggering events for episodic weakness, pain, and stiffness: during or immediately after exercise, after brief or prolonged exercise, after exercise followed by rest, after a high-carbohydrate meal, relieved by exercise, drugs/toxins, temperature (e.g., metabolic myopathies).
- Family history of myopathic disorder: X-linked, autosomal dominant, autosomal recessive, maternal transmission (mitochondrial). These conditions have a chronic presentation.
- Associated systemic symptoms/signs: rash, baldness, fever, dark red urine, dysmorphic features, cardiac, pulmonary, arthritis, other connective-tissue disease (CTD) findings, cataracts, mental retardation/dementia, skeletal contractures, skeletal deformities.

Patterns: Barohn and colleagues (2) discussed 10 patterns to identify various myopathic conditions. Some of these patterns are useful to diagnose chronic conditions; others are used to diagnose acute and subacute conditions.
- Proximal limb-girdle weakness is the most common pattern

- ▣ Acute/subacute presentation is seen with inflammatory conditions (polymyositis and dermatomyositis)—pain/rash/connective tissue disease, endocrine conditions, toxic drugs
- Distal weakness: subacute and acute presentation is seen in NMJ disease
- Proximal arm/distal leg weakness: mostly chronic muscular dystrophy, congenital myopathies, and metabolic myopathies
- Distal arm/proximal leg weakness: myotonic dystrophy and inclusion body myositis, both of which have a chronic, slowly progressive course (discussed in another chapter)
- With ocular involvement
  - ▣ Ptosis/ophthalmoplegia: Only MG has an acute/subacute presentation.
    - ○ Ptosis without ophthalmoplegia: myotonic dystrophy, congenital myopathies (chronic conditions).
    - ○ Ptosis with ophthalmoplegia: oculopharyngeal dystrophy, mitochondrial myopathy, centronuclear myopathy, neuromuscular junction disorder (MG, LEMS, botulism). Among these conditions, neuromuscular junction disorders present with subacute onset.
  - ▣ Diplopia: MG.
- Prominent neck and trunk extensor weakness: Isolated neck extensor weakness myopathy (INEM), isolated trunk extensor weakness myopathy (ITEM), MG, dermatomyositis (DM), polymyositis (PM), and inclusion body myositis (IBM). Also seen in other chronic progressive conditions, including myotonic dystrophy, fascioscapulohumeral muscular dystrophy (FSHD), congenital myopathy, carnitine deficiency, hyperparathyroidism, and overlap pattern with ALS.
- Bulbar weakness: Includes weakness of the tongue/pharyngeal/diaphragm (dysarthria or dysphagia, dyspnea). MG and LEMS may have a subacute presentation. Oculopharyngeal dystrophy, limb-girdle muscular dystrophies (LGMD) 1A myotilinopathy, myotonic dystrophy, IBM, Pompe disease, overlap pattern with ALS, and Kennedy's disease usually present as chronic progressive conditions.
- Episodic pain, weakness, rhabdomyolysis/myoglobinuria with trigger
  - ▣ Related to exercise: glycogenosis after brief exercise (e.g., McArdle's disease), lipid disorders after long exercise (carnitine palmityl transferase [CPT] deficiency), and exercise
  - ▣ Not related to exercise: malignant hyperthermia, drug/toxins, trauma(crush injury) other neuroleptic malignant syndrome, and epileptic status

- Episodic weakness delayed or unrelated to exercise
  - MG
  - Periodic paralysis: Na^+ channelopathies (hyperkalemic), Ca^{++} channelopathies (hypokalemic), Andersen's syndrome, secondary PP (thyrotoxicosis)
- Stiffness/decreased ability to relax
  - Improves with exercise: myotonia, usually Cl-channelopathy
  - Worsens with exercise/cold sensitivity: paramyotonia, Na^+ channelopathy, body's disease
  - With fixed weakness: seen in chronic conditions
    - Myotonic dystrophy (DM1)
    - Proximal myotonic dystrophy (DM2)
    - Becker's disease (autosomal recessive Cl-channelopathy)
  - Other-rippling muscle, neuromyotonia, stiff-person are also mostly chronic conditions
- Botulism: Rare serious illness caused by the botulinum toxin produced by *Clostridium botulinum*. Usually acute presentation with onset of symptoms 18 to 38 hours of exposure, but can be up to 1 week after infection. Transmission occurs through food, via contact with contaminated soil, or through an open wound. Without early treatment, botulism can lead to paralysis, breathing difficulties, and death. There are three main types: infant botulism, foodborne botulism, and wound botulism. According to the Centers for Disease Control and Prevention (CDC), about 145 cases of botulism are reported every year. Patients usually have rapidly progressive descending paralysis with dysphagia, dysarthria, ptosis, extraocular muscle weakness, mild sensory symptoms, and significant autonomic symptoms. In addition to weakness, examination shows dilated pupils, autonomic signs, and reduced tendon reflexes. Diagnosis is mainly clinical. EDX testing shows a modest increment on fast repetitive nerve stimulation (RNS) (between 40% and 100%), a decrement on slow RNS, small motor responses, on NCS and normal sensory potentials/EMG shows active denervation changes. Analysis of serum, feces, and implicated food is useful. Passive transfer of the serum or other body fluid to mice and establishing the toxicity in mice, and prevention with antitoxin, is used for definitive diagnosis. However, management should not be delayed. It includes supportive care and human trivalent antitoxin.
- Lambert-Eaton myasthenic syndrome (LEMS): Prevalence is 1 in 100,000, males are more commonly affected than females, and the age of onset is usually after 40 years (7–80 years). Onset at a younger age is seen with autoimmune LEMS,

whereas older onset cases have cancer, particularly small cell lung cancer. Weakness in the legs is present in 82% of patients, and this syndrome precedes cancer in more than 80% of patients. Legs (98%) are more affected than arms (82%). Neck weakness is seen in 82% of patients, respiratory weakness in 15%, and bulbar weakness in 22% to 56%. Other symptoms include fatigue, dysarthria, and sustained exercise. Ocular involvement is seen less often with this condition as compared to MG. Distal symmetric neuropathy is seen in few patients. Autonomic neuropathy is seen in a large percentage of patients with LEMs, including symptoms such as dry mouth, impotence, and blurred vision. On examination, proximal leg weakness is more commonly seen. This finding, when associated with paresthesias in the feet and autonomic symptoms, usually helps in diagnosing this condition. Tendon reflexes are diminished or absent at rest, but reappear after brief maximal voluntary contraction. Ataxia and encephalopathy are common in paraneoplastic LEMS. Although the ocular muscle may be affected, LEMS never begins with ocular weakness, and weakness is more prominent in the legs than in the arms. Diagnosis is based on clinical examination, elevated anti-P/Q voltage-gated calcium-channel (VGCC) antibody titers in the blood, and an increment seen on fast RNS. Notably, 15% of patients with LEMS may not have the VGCC antibodies. LEMS with neoplasm is usually associated with small cell lung cancer. Treatment includes 3,4-diaminopyridine 20 mg, immunosuppressive therapy including prednisone, cyclosporine, plasma exchange, IVIG, and treatment of the neoplasm.

- Idiopathic inflammatory myopathy: Four major categories of idiopathic inflammatory myopathy are distinguished: dermatomyositis (DM), polymyositis (PM), immune-mediated necrotizing myopathy (NM), and inclusion body myositis (IBM). Except for IBM and NM, these can occur in isolation or in association with cancer or various connective tissue diseases (overlap syndromes). The annual incidence of these disorders is approximately 1 case per 100,000 population. IBM has a slow chronic progressive course and is discussed in another chapter, whereas the other conditions present with a subacute onset and are discussed here. The age of onset for PM and NM is usually older than 18 years, whereas DM has either a childhood (juvenile) or an adulthood (adult) onset. Onset is usually subacute or insidious. The pattern of weakness is usually symmetric proximal, rather than distal, in PM and NM. In DM, PM, and NM symmetrical proximal legs are more involved than arms, and neck flexors are more diffusely involved than neck extensors. Asymmetric weakness, ocular weakness, isolated dysarthria, excludes PM, NM, and DM. Heliotrope rash,

Gottron's papules, V-sign, shawl sign, and holster signs are suggestive of DM and allow this condition to be differentiated from PM and NM. Serum creatine kinase (CK) is elevated in PM and NM, but may not be elevated in 10% of DM cases. NCS may be normal or show decreased motor amplitudes. EMG shows increased insertional and spontaneous activity in the form of fibrillation potentials, positive sharp waves, or complex repetitive discharges. Morphometric analysis reveals the presence of short-duration, small-amplitude motor unit potentials with early recruitment. Magnetic resonance imaging shows diffuse or patchy increased signaling (edema) within muscle tissue on STIR images. Myositis-specific antibodies are seen with these conditions. The Bohan and Peter criteria are used for diagnosis of PM and DM. Muscle biopsy findings in PM include endomysial inflammatory cell infiltrate (T cells) surrounding and invading non-necrotic muscle fibers, whereas perimysial inflammation and perifascicular atrophy are markers of DM. Ubiquitous major histocompatibility complex (MHC-1) expression is seen in PM diffusely and mostly in the periphery of DM. Other muscle biopsy findings associated with DM include membrane attack complex (MAC) deposition on blood vessels, reduced capillary density, myxovirus resistance 1 protein deposition on small blood vessels or muscle fibers, perivascular and tubuloreticular inclusions in endothelial walls on EM. The predominant histologic feature of the muscle biopsy in NM is presence of many necrotic fibers. The inflammatory cells are sparse or only slightly present in NM. MAC deposition on small blood vessels, pipestem capillaries on EM, no evidence of mononuclear inflammatory cells invading non-necrotic muscle fibers, and no perifascicular atrophy are seen in NM. Corticosteroids are the first-line treatment for DM, PM, and NM. Patients are started on high-dose corticosteroids and gradually tapered down. In patients who do not improve after 3 months of prednisone, are unable to taper down the steroids, or have significant corticosteroid side effects, a second-line agent (methotrexate, azathioprine, mycophenolate, IVIG, or rituximab) is used.

- Many toxic myopathies present with an acute or subacute onset. They are commonly classified based on the pathogenic mechanism triggered by the toxin—for example, necrotizing myopathy, mitochondrial myopathy, inflammatory myopathy, amphiphilic, antimicrotubular, hypokalemic, and so on. Some of the drugs that cause toxic myopathy include cholesterol-lowering agents, cyclosporine, labetalol, propofol, chloroquine, hydroxychloroquine, amiodarone, colchicine, diuretics, and corticosteroids. Predominantly proximal weakness is seen with most of these conditions. CK is usually elevated.

Muscle biopsy is useful for diagnosis. Stopping the offending agent usually leads to improvement. Progression can be seen with some of these conditions even after stopping the drug, such as statin-induced autoimmune myopathy, so immuno-suppressive therapy may be necessary.

TREATMENT

There has been a marked improvement in treatment of neuromuscular diseases because of better understanding of the pathogenic mechanisms of the conditions and extensive research and development of immunotherapies.

- Corticosteroids are the mainstay of therapy for inflammatory myopathies. Tuberculosis testing using TB quantiferon or purified protein derivative (PPD) skin test is performed prior to starting steroids. Prednisone is started at a dose of 1.5 mg/kg, up to a maximum of 100 mg per day. The dose is maintained for 2 to 4 weeks, then decreased to 100 mg every other day. For severe disease, this dose is tapered slowly over 2 to 3 months, with a 10 mg decrease every other day until a dose of 100 mg every other day is reached. Patients are maintained on the high dose for 4 to 6 months and gradually tapered by 5 to 10 mg every 2 to 3 weeks. Once the dose is decreased to 20 mg every other day, a slower taper is suggested. Second-line agents (methotrexate, azathioprine, mycophenolate mofetil, IVIG) are added for patients who do not improve significantly, who experience side effects of steroids, or who are unable to taper steroids. Rituximab may be effective, especially in patients with DM. Intravenous solumedrol 1 g daily for 3 days has also been used prior to starting oral dosing. Bone density is monitored yearly during the steroid therapy.

- Inflammatory demyelinating neuropathies: Corticosteroids are of no benefit for treatment of acute inflammatory demyelinating neuropathies and in treatment of SIDP. They are mainly used for CIDP. The American Academy of Neurology recommends plasma exchange for nonambulant adult patients with GBS who seek treatment within 4 weeks of the onset of symptoms and for ambulant patients examined within 2 weeks of the onset of symptoms (level B). IVIG is recommended for nonambulant adult patients with GBS within 2 weeks (level A) or possibly 4 weeks of the onset of neuropathic symptoms. Sequential treatment with IVIG followed by PE, or vice versa, is not indicated. In children with severe PE, IVIG or PE is a treatment option. Management of CIDP is discussed in Chapter 4.

- Motor neuron disease: Currently there are no effective treatments that can reverse or arrest the disease progression in ALS. The goal in clinical trials is to slow the disease progression to the extent possible and to help the patient maintain independent function, safety, and comfort. Education, counseling, and symptom management are important for patients with motor neuron disease. Percutaneous gastrostomy is recommended when the patient is experiencing loss of weight of more than 10% of baseline weight and doubling of eating time, and ideally is performed before the forced vital capacity falls below 50% of the predicted level. Noninvasive positive-pressure ventilation is recommended when the patient is symptomatic from shortness of breath. Symptomatic management is required to address sialorrhea (e.g., glycopyrrolate, tricyclic antidepressants, robinul), secretion clearance (e.g., cough assist devices, home suction, expectorants), pseudobulbar affect (e.g., dextromethorphan hydrobromide and quinidine sulfate, tricyclic antidepressants), depression, laryngospasm (antihistamines, antacids), neck drop (cervical collar, wheelchair with supports), communication (erasable slates, augmentative communication devices), hypoventilation (Bupa, noninvasive positive pressure ventilation [NIPPV]) contractures (e.g., night splints, botulinum toxin), foot drop (ankle foot orthotics), bed mobility (hospital bed), house accessibility (e.g., chair lift), constipation, urinary urgency, and safety. Riluzole was the first (identified in 1994) and only disease-specific treatment for a long time that was shown to positively affect the natural history of ALS. Its dose is 50 mg twice daily. There have been multiple trials with various medications performed over the years without any positive results. There are multiple ongoing trials of ALS therapies, including stem cell trials looking at neuroprotection. Edaravone (MC186), a free-radical scavenger and antioxidant, has been approved in Japan and received FDA approval in 2017.

Multifocal motor neuropathy (MMN): Patients with MMN respond to IVIG therapy. For patients who continue to progress on IVIG, rituximab may be considered. Cyclophosphamide and plasma exchange (PE) are other options to consider if there is no benefit with IVIG or rituximab.

- Neuromuscular junction disorders: MG and LEMS are the major conditions in this category.
  - Management of myasthenic crisis involves protection of the airway and management of respiratory failure. Intubation is considered at negative inspiratory force (Nif) < –20 and FVC < 1,000 mL. The details of this decision are discussed in Chapter 2. Pyridostigmine is the first-line treatment for MG. If the patient requires more than 60 mg of pyridostigmine four times per day, immunosuppressive treatment should be started. Anticholinergic medications are administered to manage side effects. Corticosteroid treatment has been the first-line immunosuppressive therapy for MG since 1970s. Improvement begins in 2 to 4 weeks; maximum benefit is seen in 6 months. Corticosteroids for MG are usually started at a high dose and gradually tapered

down. Some physicians start at a low dose and then increase the dose gradually and switch to every other day dosing. IVIG and PE are both effective treatment for MG. Other immunosuppressive medications used include azathioprine up to 2 to 3 mg/kg/day dose and cyclosporine. Mycophenolate mofetil and methotrexate trials have not produced positive results. Other emerging therapies include eculizumab, a complement inhibitor; rituximab, a monoclonal antibody to B cells; belimumab; subcutaneous immune globulin; maintenance immunoglobulin; tirasemtiv, which increases muscle contraction; and EN101 antisense oligodeoxynucleotide (Monarsen), which reduces the amount of mRNA that encodes acetylcholinesterase.

- LEMS: Treat the underlying cancer if present. 3,4-diaminopyridine blocks the outward K^+ efflux, causing increased duration of presynaptic action potential. This indirectly prolongs activation of VGCC and increases Ca^{++} entry. The dose is 10 to 20 mg three or four times per day. Guanidine hydrochloride works for some patients, but side effects restrict its use. Other immunosuppressive therapies used include prednisone, azathioprine, mycophenolate, cyclosporine, PE, and IVIG.

- Neuropathic pain is managed with antidepressants, anticonvulsants, topical agents, analgesics, and opioid drugs. Other nonpharmacologic therapies include lifestyle modification, physical therapy, podiatric care, biofeedback and relaxation therapies, acupuncture, and supplements. Controversial interventions include interventional/regional anesthesia, spinal cord neurostimulation, anodyne or monochromatic near infrared energy (MIRE) therapy, and peripheral nerve decompression.

- Autonomic dysfunction: Autonomic dysfunction is treated by addressing the symptoms. Lifestyle changes and symptomatic management is necessary. Orthostasis is managed by elevating the head of the bed, drinking enough fluids, and wearing compression stockings. Florinef, droxidopa, and midodrine are used for orthostatic hypotension. Underlying causes such as alcohol use disorder, diabetes, or Parkinson disease should be assessed and managed. If the autonomic dysfunction is due to an autoimmune process (acute pandysautonomia or acetylcholine ganglionic neuronal antibody positivity), immunosuppressive therapies may be useful.

REFERENCES

1. Oh SJ, Kurokawa K, de Almeida DF, et al. Subacute inflammatory demyelinating polyneuropathy. *Neurology.* 2003;61(11):1507–1112.

2. Barohn RJ, Dimachkie MM, Jackson CE. A pattern recognition approach to patients with a suspected myopathy. *Neurol Clin.* 2014;32(3):569–593. doi:10.1016/j.ncl.2014.04.008

SUGGESTED READING

Barohn RJ, Amato AA. Pattern-recognition approach to neuropathy and neuronopathy. *Neurol Clin.* 2013;31(2):343–361. doi:10.1016/j.ncl.2013.02.001

Chevret S, Hughes RA, Annane D. Plasma exchange for Guillain-Barré syndrome. *Cochrane Database Syst Rev.* 2017;2:CD001798. doi:10.1002/14651858.CD001798.pub3

Dimachkie MM, Barohn RJ. Motor neuron disease. *Neurol Clin.* 2015;33(4):xiii–xiv. doi:10.1016/j.ncl.2015.09.001

Pasnoor M, Barohn RJ, Dimachkie MM. Toxic myopathies. *Neurol Clin.* 2014;32(3):647–670. doi:10.1016/j.ncl.2014.04.009

Patwa HS, Chaudhry V, Katzberg H, et al. Evidence-based guideline: intravenous immunoglobulin in the treatment of neuromuscular disorders: report of the Therapeutics and Technology Assessment Subcommittee of the American Academy of Neurology. *Neurology.* 2012;78(13):1009–1015. doi:10.1212/WNL.0b013e31824de293

William W. Campbell. *Dejong's The Neurologic Examination.* Philadelphia, PA: Lippincott Williams and Wilkins; 2005.

4 Chronically Developing Weakness

Hans D. Katzberg, Ari Breiner, and Aaron Izenberg

HISTORY

- When considering a patient with chronically developing weakness, one would like to ascertain the age of onset of symptoms, the rate of progression, the distribution of weakness, and any associated systemic features that may help to narrow the differential diagnosis.

- First, however, the clinician should ensure that the patient is truly describing *weakness*, rather than a mimicking condition. For example, rheumatologic disease (such as rheumatoid arthritis or fibromyalgia) may cause myalgias/arthralgias that are interpreted as weakness; and metabolic/endocrine conditions (including electrolyte abnormalities) or other medical diseases (including cardiac or renal failure) may cause generalized fatigue and exercise intolerance that could be viewed as weakness by the patient. To prove that the patient has true neurologic weakness, it is helpful to ask questions regarding typical daily activities—including pattern of gait, falls, stair climbing, using keys and utensils, and reaching above one's head.

- It is of critical importance to determine whether the patient is experiencing sensory symptoms or fluctuations. The presence of even subtle sensory symptoms could implicate localizations such as the cerebral cortex or spinal cord, peripheral nerves, plexi, or nerve roots.

- The presence of fatigability or fluctuation may suggest the presence of a neuromuscular junction disorder. Conversely, if a true, progressive pure motor syndrome is identified, this may help to narrow the differential diagnosis to disorders affecting the muscle, neuromuscular junction, motor nerves, or anterior horn cells.

- The pattern of weakness can be clarified during history taking and will help to narrow the differential diagnosis.

    - A length-dependent, distal-to-proximal pattern of weakness might be associated with a motor-predominant polyneuropathy, although myopathies, polyradiculopathies, and motor neuron diseases may also present with distal-predominant weakness (albeit less commonly). The differential diagnosis of distally predominant myopathy is discussed later in this chapter.

■ Similarly, a proximal pattern of weakness would best localize to the muscle, although neuromuscular junction and motor neuron disease, as well as polyradiculopathy, may cause proximal weakness.

■ Other patterns to explore on history would include ocular or bulbar presentations, diaphragmatic weakness, axial weakness, focal weakness (affecting a single peripheral nerve, root, or limb), or multifocal weakness.

- The patient's family history is helpful to distinguish inherited from acquired neuromuscular conditions. In cases where other family members are affected, a full pedigree should be constructed, to determine whether the pattern of inheritance is most consistent with dominant, recessive, X-linked, or maternal transmission. Even when family members are unaffected, a recessively transmitted condition or a *de novo* mutation should still be considered. Affected family members may be unaware of the presence of neuromuscular disease, particularly in milder or very slowly progressive conditions. For example, many cases of hereditary motor and sensory neuropathy (Charcot-Marie-Tooth disease) and mitochondrial myopathies have been recognized only after the examination of supposedly unaffected family members.

- A history of medication use, social history, toxic ingestions, and developmental milestones should also be reviewed.

- In addition to characterization of weakness, associated symptoms are helpful to narrow the differential diagnosis. Muscle cramps, atrophy, and fasciculations are more suggestive of a neurogenic condition, whereas muscle pseudohypertrophy, contractures, or cardiac involvement are more suggestive of myopathy.

- The findings on systemic review will relate to the underlying condition—for example, patients with myotonic dystrophy may report the presence of cataracts and diabetes, temporal muscle atrophy, and difficulty releasing a hand grip. The presence of progressive weakness with episodic myoglobinuria (pigmented urine) might suggest an underlying muscular dystrophy or metabolic myopathy. As a result, a complete history and full review of systems is recommended.

INVESTIGATIONS IN CHRONICALLY DEVELOPING WEAKNESS

Physical Examination

1. Inspection: Overall inspection of the patient should be performed looking for the presence of joint contractures, scoliosis, bony deformities such as pes cavus or pectum excavatum, and skin

rash (e.g., heliotrope rash or shawl sign in dermatomyositis). The presence of respiratory muscles weakness (including accessory muscle use or paradoxical chest movement) should be observed. The pattern of gait should be noted as the patient enters the examination room. General inspection may reveal an obvious pattern of muscle atrophy, hypertrophy, or the presence of fasciculations.

2. Cognitive examination: A screening cognitive examination may be abnormal in patients with selected hereditary causes of chronically progressive weakness, including myotonic dystrophy, congenital myopathies, leukodystrophies, and mitochondrial disorders, among others. We recommend using a standardized test (such as the Folstein Mini-Mental Status Examination [MMSE] or the Montreal Cognitive Examination [MoCA]) to allow comparison with normative values.

3. Cranial nerve examination: The cranial nerve examination should focus on the presence of extraocular muscle weakness, ptosis, or facial weakness. The presence of facial weakness may result in a horizontal smile, inability to bury the eyelashes, or difficulty maintaining a lip seal. The presence of tongue atrophy or fasciculations, and a brisk jaw-jerk reflex may indicate the presence of a motor neuron disease. The patient's speech should be evaluated to determine whether a spastic or flaccid pattern of dysarthria is present.

4. Motor examination: Muscle bulk and the presence of fasciculations should be commented upon after careful observation of muscles at rest, with individual muscles uncovered and appropriate draping used to preserve patient privacy. Tone should be examined in a relaxed patient, in the supine position. The presence of spasticity in the setting of atrophy and other lower motor neuron signs may be suggestive of a motor neuron disease. Reduced muscle tone (hypotonia) may be observed in children, but is difficult to distinguish from normal tone in the adult patient. The pattern and degree of muscle weakness according to the Medical Research Council scale should be recorded. This should include examination of the neck flexor and extensor muscles, which could indirectly give some indication of diaphragmatic strength. Special tests include inspection for the presence of scapular winging, tests of percussion and grip myotonia (demonstrating delayed muscle relaxation), performance of squats for detection of subtle hip-girdle weakness, and Gower's sign. Upright and supine FVC done portably in the neuromuscular clinic could also give useful information about diaphragmatic function.

5. Reflexes: Reflexes should be graded as normal (2+), pathologically brisk (3+ or 4+ if sustained clonus), hypoactive (1+), or absent. The measurement of reflexes will help to determine whether the weakness is of an upper or lower motor neuron type, and the degree of symmetry of the process.

6. Sensory examination: In a pure motor syndrome, both large- and small-fiber sensory modalities should be within normal limits. If sensory symptoms and signs predominate, then the patient most likely has a primary disorder of the peripheral nerves or nerve roots, which are addressed in a separate chapter of this book. However, some patients with chronically progressive weakness may have motor-predominant, rather than motor-exclusive, syndromes. Therefore, a careful examination of pinprick, temperature sensation, proprioception, and vibration thresholds is important. The presence of a fixed sensory level should not be missed, and suggests localization to the spinal cord, rather than a neuromuscular cause of weakness. For measurement of vibration, the authors prefer quantitative methods, which would include either the Rydel-Seiffer tuning fork or a biothesiometer. Using these methods, vibration thresholds can be compared at subsequent visits.

7. Gait: Patients with chronic weakness may have a waddling gait (suggestive of proximal muscle weakness), foot slap (suggestive of distal weakness), or a spastic gait with circumduction. Some patients may be unable to ambulate independently and may require ankle orthotics, or a cane, walker, or wheelchair. In ambulatory patients, time- or distance-based tests (such as the timed get-up-and-go or 6-minute walk test) may be helpful for longitudinal evaluation, or to determine the response to treatment.

Paraclinical Investigations

Selection of diagnostic investigations for a patient with chronically progressive weakness should follow from the information provided from the history and examination. If the patient has a true, pure motor syndrome, the differential diagnosis is more focused on myopathy, disorders of neuromuscular transmission, motor neuron diseases, and the rare causes of pure motor neuropathy. However, if the patient has even subtle sensory symptoms or exam findings, the possible localization expands considerably to include peripheral neuropathy, radicular disease, and pathology at the level of the spinal cord or brain.

Electrophysiology

Electrodiagnostic testing is indispensible in the workup of any patient with a suspected neuromuscular cause of weakness. Conventional testing involves nerve conduction studies (NCS) and needle electromyography (EMG).

- In NCS, sensory nerve action potentials (SNAPs) are recorded from the skin superficial to the nerve, and compound motor action potentials (CMAPs) are recorded off of a muscle innervated by the nerve of interest. NCS are typically most informative in neurogenic disorders, although abnormalities can also be seen in myopathies and disorders of neuromuscular transmission.

In patients with pure motor syndromes (i.e., myopathy, neuro-muscular junction [NMJ] disease, and motor neuron diseases), one may see a pattern of attenuated or unobtainable CMAPs, with relatively spared SNAPs. NCS can also be quite helpful to dis-tinguish between demyelinating and axonal neuropathies, both of which may cause of chronic weakness. In demyelinating neu-ropathies such as hereditary motor sensory neuropathy (HMSN), multifocal motor neuropathy (MMN), and chronic inflammatory demyelinating polyneuropathy (CIDP) responses often have slowed conduction velocities, plus prolonged distal latencies and minimal F-wave latencies, with conduction block present in acquired conditions. Conversely, axonal neuropathies are charac-terized more by reduced response amplitudes, with relative pres-ervation of velocity and latency.

- Needle EMG involves insertion of a needle electrode directly into the muscle. The muscle is examined at rest to assess for abnor-mal insertional and spontaneous activity. Fibrillation potentials and positive sharp waves are seen in neurogenic conditions with active/uncompensated denervation, and in myopathies with necrosis, splitting, or inflammation. Other forms of abnormal spontaneous activity include cramp and fasciculation potentials, which are seen in neurogenic and benign/physiological states; complex repetitive discharges, which are seen in very chronic myopathic and neurogenic disorders; and myotonic discharges, which are seen most classically in myotonic dystrophies and non-dystrophic myotonias. Table 4.1 summarizes the common needle EMG findings in a variety of neuromuscular disorders.

- Repetitive nerve stimulation (RNS) is used in the diagnosis of diagnosis of myasthenia gravis (MG) and other NMJ disorders. In MG, 2–3 Hz RNS will often reveal an electrodecrement of 10% or more. Repeating this test after 10–15 seconds of exercise will often reveal improvement—a phenomenon referred to as post-exercise

TABLE 4.1 Common Needle EMG Findings

	Spontaneous activity	Voluntary activity
Neurogenic disease	• Fibrillation potentials and positive sharp waves (if active denervation) • Fasciculation potentials • Cramp potentials	• MUAPs with increased amplitude and duration (if chronic denervation) • Decreased recruitment pattern
Myopathy	• Fibrillation potentials and positive sharp waves (in some conditions) • Myotonic discharges (e.g., myotonic dystrophy)	• MUAPs with decreased (increased) amplitude and duration • Early recruitment pattern

MUAP, motor unit action potential.

repair. Higher-frequency RNS at 30–50 Hz can reveal an incremental response of more than 100% in Lambert-Eaton myasthenic syndrome (LEMS), although the high-frequency stimulation has largely been replaced with 10 seconds of maximal exercise (the high-frequency stimulation is often painful).

- Single fiber EMG (SFEMG) is another specialized study used in the investigation of NMJ disorders. The classic abnormality seen is increased "jitter," a measurement of the variability of the time interval between a pair of multiple muscle fiber action potentials originating from the same motor unit. Intermittent blocking of these potentials can also be seen.

Laboratory Investigations

- A basic screen for a length-dependent sensorimotor axonal polyneuropathy should include assessment for diabetes (HbA1c) as well as vitamin B_{12} level, serum protein electrophoresis, and immunofixation. For multifocal and severe, rapidly progressing neuropathies, a more expanded set of lab investigations should be included to assess for autoimmune diseases (including vasculitis), infectious diseases, and paraneoplastic causes. Assessment of specific autoantibodies can be requested when there is suspicion for an immune-mediated neuropathy (e.g., anti-GM1 in MMN, or anti-GD1a in acute motor axonal neuropathy).

  In the setting of a suspected myopathy, serum creatine kinase (CK) should be tested, as well as lactate and thyroid-stimulating hormone (TSH). Additional myositis-specific autoantibodies can be assessed when there is suspicion for an immune-mediated myopathy. Patients with possible MG should have acetylcholine receptor antibody (AChRAb) titers drawn. If this is normal in a case of generalized myasthenia gravis, and there is persistent suspicion for MG, anti-muscle-specific kinase (MuSK) and LRP4 antibodies can also be sent.

- A lumbar puncture (LP) should be considered when there is concern for an immune-mediated polyradiculoneuropathy. In CIDP (as with Guillain-Barré syndrome [GBS]) one often sees a characteristic pattern of cytoalbuminological dissociation—that is, elevated cerebrospinal fluid (CSF) protein with normal white blood cell (WBC) count. An LP with cell count, cytology, and flow cytometry should also be performed if there is a concern for an infiltrative or neoplastic polyradiculopathy.

- Genetic testing can be arranged in patients with suspected hereditary neuropathies (e.g., Charcot-Marie-Tooth [CMT] disease, hereditary motor neuropathies [HMN]) and myopathies (muscular dystrophies, congenital myopathies, channelopathies, and metabolic/mitochondrial diseases). Table 4.2 identifies suggested lab testing in different clinical presentations.

TABLE 4.2 Suggested Laboratory Investigations in Neuromuscular Disease

Suspected disease	Investigations
Length-dependent peripheral neuropathy	• HbA1c • Vitamin B$_{12}$ • SPEP and immunofixation
Multifocal and/or acute neuropathy	• ANA, ENA panel, ESR, CRP, RF, ACE • ANCAs, C3/C4, cryoglobulin screen • HIV, syphilis, Lyme disease, HCV, and HBV serologies *Also consider depending on clinical context:* • Lumbar puncture • Heavy metal screen (e.g., mercury, lead, arsenic) • GM1 antibodies (and antibodies to other gangliosides • Paraneoplastic antibodies • WNV serology • Porphyria screen • Genetic testing (e.g., CMT, HMN)
Myopathy	• CK • TSH • Liver function tests • Myositis-specific antibodies *(in suspected immune-mediated myopathies)* • Genetic testing *(in suspected hereditary myopathies)*
Motor neuron disease	• CK • SPEP and immunofixation • Lyme disease serology *In pure lower motor neuron presentations consider adding:* • GM1 antibodies • WNV serology • Heavy metal screen *In pure upper motor neuron presentations consider adding:* • Vitamin E • Serum copper • Syphilis screen

(continued)

TABLE 4.2 Suggested Laboratory Investigations in Neuromuscular Disease (*continued*)

Suspected disease	Investigations
Neuromuscular junction disease	• AChR antibodies • MuSK and LRP4 antibodies • P/Q-type voltage-gated potassium antibodies *(in suspected LEMS)* • Stool for botulinum toxin *(in suspected botulism)*

ACE, angiotensin converting enzyme; AchR, acetylcholine receptor; ANA, antinuclear antibody; ANCA, anti-neutrophil cytoplasmic antibody; CK, creatine kinase; CMT, Charcot-Marie-Tooth disease; CRP, C-reactive protein; ENA, encapsulated nuclear antibody; ESR, erythrocyte sedimentation rate; HBV, hepatitis B virus; HCV, hepatitis C virus; HMN, hereditary motor neuropathies; LEMS, Lambert-Eaton myasthenic syndrome; LRP4, lipoprotein receptor–related protein 4; MuSK, muscle-specifi c tyrosine kinase; RF, rheumatoid factor; SPEP, serum protein electrophoresis; TSH, thyroid-stimulating hormone; WNV, West Nile virus.

PATHOLOGICAL STUDIES

Although many hereditary conditions can be diagnosed through genetic testing, muscle biopsy still serves a central role in the investigation of many myopathies. Muscle tissue can be analyzed through a variety of histochemical and immunohistochemical stains, electron microscopy, and molecular studies.

• Myopathies reveal a wide variety of histopathological findings, though some basic patterns can be identified. Nonspecific myopathic findings include atrophic fibers, varied muscle fiber size, and fiber splitting. The myositides are often associated with inflammatory cell infiltrates of varying distribution depending on the disease subtype. A characteristic finding in muscular dystrophies is increased endomysial connective tissue. Many toxic myopathies are associated with muscle fiber necrosis and phagocytosis.

• Nerve biopsies can be very useful in selected circumstances, though they are done much less frequently today due to the potential for significant morbidity, and the increasing ability to diagnose neuropathies by other means. Nerve biopsy may be a consideration in the setting of a severe neuropathy with an otherwise unrevealing, complete workup. This approach is often pursued when there is concern for nonsystemic vasculitic neuropathy or amyloidosis (familial or sporadic).

IMAGING

As noted earlier, though pure motor weakness is most commonly seen in neuromuscular disorders, it is important to exclude structural disease of the brain and spinal cord using imaging techniques. In patients with limb weakness, magnetic resonance imaging (MRI) of the relevant level(s) of the spinal cord is often indicated, and in the setting of bulbar weakness a brain MRI should be performed to exclude brainstem disease.

Nerve and muscle imaging are also being used more frequently in patients with neuromuscular disease. Muscle MRI can reveal areas of inflammation and edema, fatty replacement, and fibrosis. This modality can provide information about disease activity and pattern of muscle involvement, and can aid in the selection of a muscle for biopsy. MR imaging can also provide important information in neurogenic conditions, including evidence of focal compression or entrapment, nerve sheath tumors, and areas of nerve inflammation.

DIFFERENTIAL DIAGNOSIS OF CHRONICALLY DEVELOPING WEAKNESS

The differential diagnosis of symmetrical, motor-exclusive weakness is presented in Table 4.3. Both neuropathic and myopathic processes can present symmetrically, and as such can be difficult to distinguish on clinical grounds alone.

TABLE 4.3 Symmetric Pure Motor Neuromuscular Syndromes

Neuropathic		
Spinal muscular atrophy (SMA types 1–4 and distal SMA)	Spinobulbar muscular atrophy (SBMA or Kennedy's disease)	GM2 gangliosidosis (Sandhoff's disease)
Isaac's syndrome (neuromyotonia)	Hereditary motor neuropathies (HMN 1–8)	Algrove's syndrome
Machado Joseph disease (spinocerebellar atrophy type 3)	Polyglucosan disease	Mitochondrial neurogastrointestinal encephalopathy (MNGIE)
Paraneoplastic motor neuropathy (breast cancer, lymphoma)	Porphyria and Refsum's neuropathies	Toxic neuropathies (lead, dapsone, botulism, tick paralysis, HIV, West Nile virus)
Myopathic		
Amyotrophic lateral sclerosis (ALS; commonly presents asymmetrically but symmetric axial, appendicular, or bulbar motor weakness can also occur)		
Guillan-Barré syndrome (rapidly progressive weakness, usually symmetric, can also have cranial nerve involvement, sensory findings, and autonomic dysfunction)		

(*continued*)

TABLE 4.3 Symmetric Pure Motor Neuromuscular Syndromes (*continued*)

Myopathic		
Dystrophinopathies (Becker and Duchenne)	Myotonic dystrophies type 1 and 2	Proximal myotonic myopathy (PROMM)
Limb-girdle muscular dystrophies 1 (autosomal dominant), 2 (autosomal recessive), X-linked (Barth syndrome, Emery-Dreifuss, and Danon disease)	Nondystrophic myotonias (myotonia congenita, paramyotonia congenita, potassium-aggravated myotonia, Schwartz-Jampel syndrome)	Inflammatory myopathies (polymyositis, dermatomyositis, inclusion body myositis), HMG-CoA reductase–associated necrotizing myopathy
Myofibrillary myopathies (types 1–8)	Collagen type 6 myopathies (Bethlem and Ulrich myopathies)	Endocrine myopathies (thyroid, adrenal dysfunction, and acromegaly)
Congenital myopathies (core, centronuclear, nemaline myopathies, congenital fiber-type disproportion)		
Metabolic myopathies (can present with episodic weakness, but can also present with progressive weakness and include glycogen storage diseases, such as Pompe disease, McArdle disease, and lipid metabolic disorders such as carnitine palmitoyl transferase deficiency)		
Toxic myopathies (statins, fibrates, steroids, antiretrovirals, chloroquine, neuromuscular blockers, amiodarone, L-tryptophan, alfa-interferon, cyclosporine, tacrolimus, labetolol, vincristine, penicillamine, cimetidine, finasteride, imatinib, omeprazole, alcohol, propofol, dehydroemetine, phenytoin, lamotrigine)		
Spinal		
Familial spinal cord syndromes and hereditary spastic paraplegia (HSP)		

- Neuropathic conditions may more commonly cause symptoms such as muscle cramps and reveal hyporeflexia on examination. Most diffuse, symmetric, pure motor neuropathic syndromes occur insidiously or at an early age and are due to inherited diseases of the motor neuron, including spinal muscular atrophy, spinobulbar muscular atrophy (Kennedy's disease), hereditary motor neuropathies (HMN), and metabolic syndromes such as GM2 gangliosidosis (Sandhoff's disease).
- Myopathic causes of diffuse symmetric weakness are more common than neuropathic ones.
  - These include congenital myopathies (inherited skeletal muscle diseases associated with early infantile or childhood onset and a static or slowly progressive course) and muscular dystrophies

(which cause a more progressive myopathy and simultaneous degeneration and regeneration of muscle tissue).

▣ Muscular dystrophies may present with a limb-girdle pattern of weakness or have unique phenotypes. For example, oculopharyngeal muscular dystrophy (OPMD) involves ocular and bulbar musculature, in addition to a limb-girdle myopathic weakness. An important associated symptom to consider in those patients presenting with myopathy is cardiac involvement, which can include cardiomyopathy and arrhythmias (Table 4.4). Although less common, myopathies can also present with a distal-predominant pattern of weakness, with selective involvement of the upper or lower extremities. The most common distal myopathies are listed in Table 4.5.

▣ Although acquired myopathies typically present in an acute fashion, they should also be considered in a patient with chronic, unexplained weakness, as the diagnosis may have been missed. The most important acquired myopathies for the clinician include toxic myopathies (due to statins, corticosteroids, or other medications) and inflammatory myopathies including dermatomyositis, polymyositis, and inclusion body myositis (IBM). More recently, a relationship has been described between certain toxic agents and inflammatory myopathy, known as necrotizing immune myopathy with antibodies to HMG-CoA reductase inhibitors (i.e., statins).

TABLE 4.4 Myopathies With Prominent Cardiac Involvement

Cardiomyopathies	Arrhythmias
Dystrophinopathies (Duchenne and Becker muscular dystrophy)	Dystrophinopathies (Duchenne and Becker muscular dystrophy)
Limb-girdle muscular dystrophy, types 1A-B, 2C-G, 2I	Limb-girdle muscular dystrophy, types 1B, 2C-G, 2I
Myotonic dystrophy	Myotonic dystrophy
Emery-Dreifuss muscular dystrophy	Emery-Dreifuss muscular dystrophy
Polymyositis	Polymyositis
Nemaline myopathy	Mitochondrial myopathy (Kearns-Sayre syndrome)
Myofibrillar myopathies	Andersen-Tawil syndrome
Acid maltase deficiency (in children)	
Carnitine deficiency	
Amyloid myopathy	

TABLE 4.5 Distally Predominant Myopathies

Inclusion body myositis (IBM)
Fascioscapulohumeral dystrophy (tibialis anterior)
Myotonic dystrophy type 1
Miyoshi's myopathy (dysferlinopathy)
Anoctamin-5 (ANO5) myopathy
LGMD1A (myotilinopathy)
LGMD1G (HNRPDL proteinopathy)
Selected congenital myopathies (late-onset nemaline myopathy, nebulin mutation)
Distal myopathy types 1–3
LGMD1A, limb-girdle muscular dystrophy type 1A; LGMD1G, limb-girdle muscular dystrophy type 1G.

- Endocrinopathies including disorders of the thyroid and adrenal axis have been associated with chronically progressive myopathy. However, other systemic findings are expected on the history and physical examination (e.g., hair loss, cold intolerance, deepened voice, and "hung" deep tendon reflexes, in advanced hypothyroidism).

- Although chronic weakness may be present in metabolic myopathies, congenital diseases of the neuromuscular junction, and channelopathies, these diseases are most often characterized by prominent fluctuations or variability, and are discussed in a separate chapter.

- Asymmetrical pure motor syndromes (Table 4.6) can comprise neuropathic and myopathic conditions, but in this situation neuropathic conditions predominate. The two main neuropathic conditions to consider are multifocal motor neuropathy (MMN) and amyotrophic lateral sclerosis (ALS). These may prove challenging to differentiate (Table 4.7), although on examination, one would expect upper motor neuron signs in ALS, including hyperreflexia, extensor plantar responses, and clonus. However, it is important to recall that there are variants of motor neuron disease that lack upper motor neuron findings, as seen in progressive muscular atrophy (PMA). In addition, one must recall that ALS can have a symmetrical onset or present in a regional manner, affecting the bulbar, axial, or respiratory muscles. MMN is also more commonly a chronic, insidious condition, whereas a key feature of ALS is a more aggressive progression and deterioration. Another, more subtle distinguishing feature is the myotomal pattern of dysfunction characteristic of ALS, in contrast to the selective motor nerve involvement in MMN.

TABLE 4.6 Asymmetric Pure Motor Neuromuscular Syndromes

Neuropathic		
Multifocal motor neuropathy (MMN) and variants (multifocal axonal motor axonopathy [MAMA])	Amyotrophic lateral sclerosis and variants (progressive muscular atrophy, primary lateral sclerosis, isolated bulbar ALS, bibrachial amyotrophic diplegia)	Monomelic amyotrophy (Hirayama's disease)
Postpolio syndrome	Chronic neuralgic amyotrophy of the brachial or lumbosacral plexus (HNA2)	Radiation plexopathy
Myopathic		
Fascioscapulohumeral dystrophy	McLeod syndrome	Inclusion body myositis
Carriers of dystrophinopathies or centronuclear myopathy	Some acid maltase (Pompe disease) and phosphorylase (McArdle's disease) deficiencies	Neutral lipid storage disease
Limb-girdle muscular dystrophy 1C (caveolinopathy), 2A (calpainopathy), 2B (miyoshi myopathy or dysferlinopathy), 2I (FKRP), 2L (anoctaminopathy)		

- A careful history should be taken to assess whether the patient experienced weakness in a limb or limbs as a neonate or child, as progressive weakness in the remotely affected limb could represent postpolio syndrome. A teenager with stationary stage after progressive arm weakness should be evaluated for monomelic

TABLE 4.7 Clinical Characteristics Distinguishing MMN From ALS

	ALS	MMN
Reflexes	Hyperreflexia	Hyporeflexia
Tone	Spastic	Normal
Bulbar findings	Often present	Absent
Pattern of weakness	Myotomal	Selected motor nerve involvement
Clinical course	Rapid/subacute	Chronic
Pseudobulbar affect	Yes	No
Cognitive involvement	Associated with frontotemporal dementia	No
Respiratory involvement	Common	Uncommon
ALS, amyotrophic lateral sclerosis; MMN, multifocal motor neuropathy.		

amyotrophy, also known as Hirayama's disease—a type of cervical myelopathy related to flexion movements of the neck. Although most myopathic conditions present with proximal, symmetric weakness as described earlier, some can present in an asymmetric manner, including fascioscapulohumeral muscular dystrophy (FSHD) and limb-girdle muscular dystrophy 2L (anoctominopathy).

- Apart from the exclusively motor syndromes, a number of neurogenic conditions present with predominantly motor involvement, although mild sensory findings are present. For example, Charcot-Marie-Tooth (CMT) disease most commonly presents with progressive weakness, usually in a distal, length-dependent fashion. However, sensory involvement is often noted on examination. Similarly, motor-predominant CIDP can present primarily with areflexia as well as proximal and distal weakness, but subtle sensory findings are typically noted on examination, including impaired vibration thresholds, or even length-dependent small-fiber sensory loss. Other predominantly motor neuropathies may include paraproteinemic neuropathies, neuropathies related to plasma cell dyscrasias, and porphyric neuropathy.

- Acquired pure motor neuropathies are rare and tend to present less insidiously than the inherited conditions. Nevertheless, toxic, inflammatory, and infectious motor neuropathies have been described and should be considered. If a patient presents with primarily spasticity and upper motor neuron signs on examination, familial spinal cord syndromes should be considered, which include the hereditary spastic paraplegias (HSP).

TREATMENT OF CHRONICALLY DEVELOPING WEAKNESS

- Most hereditary neuropathies and myopathies mentioned in this chapter have limited disease-modifying treatment options. Research endeavors evaluating gene therapy and other treatments for inherited neuropathic conditions and muscular dystrophies are ongoing, and encouraging clinical trials of therapy with antisense oligonucleotide therapy for children with spinal muscular atrophy and exon skipping therapy in children with Duchenne muscular dystrophy and selected gene mutations have been completed.

- Similarly, metabolic myopathies have limited treatment options, but enzyme replacement for acid maltase deficiency, also known as Pompe disease, has been shown to improve respiratory and motor outcomes.

- Certain patients with congenital myopathies have been reported to experience benefits from acetylcholinesterase inhibitors in centronuclear myopathies and albuterol in core myopathies.

- In certain myopathies where the inflammatory process is thought to contribute to weakness and disability, such as in ambulatory boys with Duchenne muscular dystrophy, limited periods of treatment with steroids including prednisone and deflazacort have been shown to extend the duration of ambulation. Vitamin and nutrient therapy including coenzyme Q10 have shown modest improvements in patients with mitochondrial disease and have evidence supporting their use in this and other metabolic myopathies.

- Treatment of acquired neuromuscular conditions presenting with chronically developing weakness depends on correcting the underlying cause, toxicity, deficiency, or pathological process. Immune myopathies such as polymyositis, dermatomyositis, and immune neuropathies including CIDP and MMN are often responsive to immunosuppression with agents such as oral or intravenous steroids and steroid-sparing agents including azathioprine, mycophenolate mofetil, methotrexate, and immunomodulation therapy with intravenous immunoglobulin (IVIG) and plasmapheresis. The response of each individual condition to a particular agent is variable; for example, patients with MMN response to steroids compared to myositis and CIDP. For some acquired conditions, few treatments have been shown to significantly alter the disease course. This includes inclusion body myositis, for which immunotherapy similar to that used in dermatomyositis and polymyositis has not proved helpful to date. As with many of the hereditary conditions, clinical trials in this area are ongoing.

- Patients with ALS also have limited treatment options. Riluzole has been shown to reduce glutamate in animal models and patients with ALS, and has been shown to offer a modest improvement in life expectancy—on average, 3 months. Edaravone is a free radical scavenger that was recently shown to slow the decline in the ALS Functional Rating Scale (ALSFRS-R), in a subset of patients with mild respiratory involvement (FVC > 80%) and a specific pattern of early progression. It is administered intravenously for 14 consecutive days in the first cycle, followed by 10-day treatment cycle with 14 drug-free days in between. Supportive care provided through multidisciplinary clinics where noninvasive ventilation, feeding tubes, and additional nutritional support are addressed has been shown to improve outcomes and also has a positive effect on life expectancy.

SUGGESTED READING

Grunseich C, Fischbeck KH. Spinal and bulbar muscular atrophy. *Neurol Clin.* 2015;33(4):847–854.

Hanewinckel R, Ikram MA, Van Doorn PA. Peripheral neuropathies. *Handb Clin Neurol.* 2016;138:263–282.

Mammen AL. Autoimmune myopathies. *Continuum (Minneap Minn)*. 2016;22(6, Muscle and Neuromuscular Junction Disorders):1852–1870.

Miller RG, Jackson CE, Kasarskis EJ, et al. Practice parameter update: the care of the patient with amyotrophic lateral sclerosis: multidisciplinary care, symptom management, and cognitive/behavioral impairment (an evidence-based review): report of the Quality Standards Subcommittee of the American Academy of Neurology. *Neurology*. 2009;73(15):1227–1233.

Mul K, Lassche S, Voermans NC, et al. What's in a name? The clinical features of facioscapulohumeral muscular dystrophy. *Pract Neurol*. 2016;16(3):201–207.

Shaibani A. Distal myopathies: case studies. *Neurol Clin*. 2016;34(3):547–564.

Smith CA, Gutmann L. Myotonic dystrophy type 1 management and therapeutics. *Curr Treat Options Neurol*. 2016;18(12):52.

Tarnopolsky MA. Metabolic myopathies. *Continuum (Minneap Minn)*. 2016:1829–1851.

Wicklund MP, Kissel JT. The limb-girdle muscular dystrophies. *Neurol Clin*. 2014;32(3):729–749.

5 Episodic Weakness and Exercise Intolerance

Carolina Barnett and Charles Kassardjian

Some neuromuscular diseases present with recurrent episodes of weakness, as opposed to chronic or slowly progressive weakness. Additionally, some neuromuscular disorders present as exercise intolerance with or without weakness.

In this chapter, we discuss the different ways that episodic weakness and exercise intolerance might manifest, as well as which findings on the physical, electrodiagnostic, and other assessments can point to different etiologies. Based on the differential diagnoses, we discuss general treatment principles for the different causes of episodic weakness and exercise intolerance.

CLINICAL MANIFESTATIONS

Episodic Weakness

An in-depth clinical history provides invaluable information to help identify the cause of the episodic weakness. The main aspects to consider are the triggers for the weakness, the duration and frequency of episodes, the anatomic distribution, the symptoms between episodes, and other accompanying symptoms. These aspects are also summarized in Table 5.1.

1. **Triggers:** These can be related to meals, exercise, weather, medication, and other illnesses.

   - Meals: Weakness triggered by a meal heavy in carbohydrates suggests a glycogen storage disease or hypokalemic periodic paralysis (PP); weakness triggered by a meal rich in potassium suggests hyperkalemic PP. Alcohol intake can trigger weakness in hypokalemic PP. Weakness triggered by fasting can be seen in fatty acid oxidation disorders as well as in hyperkalemic PP. Fasting or a diet low in carbohydrates can trigger a porphyria attack.

   - Exercise: Weakness triggered by intense physical activity followed by a period of rest suggests PP, whereas weakness that occurs with exercise and that improves with rest may occur

TABLE 5.1 Clinical Characteristics of Episodic Weakness and/or Exercise Intolerance Caused by Different Diseases

Triggers	Hypokalemic PP	Hyperkalemic PP	MG	Glycogen storage disorders	Fatty acid oxidation disorders	Recurrent rhabdomyolysis (not metabolic myopathy)	HNPP	Acute intermittent porphyria
Exercise trigger	Rest after exercise	Rest after exercise	During or right after exercise, better with rest	Triggered by intense, brief exercise. "Second wind" in McArdle's disease.	Sustained exercise	Intense or sustained exercise	No	No
Meals trigger	Meal high in carbohydrates or alcohol	Meal high in potassium or fasting	No effect	Meal high in carbohydrates	Fasting	No	No	Fasting or low in carbohydrates, alcohol
Temperature trigger	None	Triggered by cold	Heat might make weakness worse	No effect	Heat or cold	No	No	No
Duration	Hours to days	Hours	Hours to days or longer	Hours	Hours	Hours to days	Hours, days or longer	Days to weeks
Medication triggers	Diuretics, insulin, intravenous glucose	K⁺-sparing diuretics	Aminoglycosides, muscle relaxants, benzodiazepines, occasionally corticosteroids (and many others)	No	General anesthesia (CPT2)	Anesthetics (malignant hyperthermia in some cases)	No	Barbiturates, oral contraceptives, benzodiazepines

(continued)

TABLE 5.1 Clinical Characteristics of Episodic Weakness and/or Exercise Intolerance Caused by Different Diseases (*continued*)

	Hypokalemic PP	Hyperkalemic PP	MG	Glycogen storage disorders	Fatty acid oxidation disorders	Recurrent rhabdomyolysis (not metabolic myopathy)	HNPP	Acute intermittent porphyria
Other symptoms/ signs								
Bulbar/ respiratory symptoms	Rare	Rare	Frequent	No	No	Generally not, but depends on the individual gene mutation	No	Yes
Extraocular muscles involvement	No	No	Frequent	No	No	No	No	Yes
Sensory changes	No	No	No	No	No	No	Can be present	Usually mild
Reflexes	Reduced or absent during attack; normal between attacks	Reduced during attacks; normal between attacks	Normal	Normal	Normal	Normal	Normal or reduced	Normal or reduced
Myotonia or paramyotonia	No	Can be present	No	No	No	No	No	No

CPT2, Carnitine palmityl transferase type 2; HNPP, hereditary neuropathy with liability to pressure palsies; MG, myasthenia gravis; PP, periodic paralysis.

in myasthenia gravis (MG). Intense exercise can also trigger recurrent rhabdomyolysis and weakness in patients with metabolic myopathies and myopathies associated with mutations of the ryanodine receptor.

- Time of day: PPs tend to occur more in the mornings (after a night's rest), whereas patients with MG tend to be better or asymptomatic upon awakening but become weak or symptomatic as the day goes by.
- Temperature: Patients with hyperkalemic PP can have weakness triggered by cold. Patients with MG often feel weaker with heat and better with cold, as cold can improve neuromuscular junction (NMJ) transmission.
- Medications: Insulin, intravenous glucose, corticosteroids, and diuretics can trigger hypokalemic PP. Potassium-sparing diuretics can trigger hyperkalemic PP. Weakness in MG can be triggered by aminoglycosides, by muscle relaxants, and in some patients who are starting corticosteroids (usually within the first 14 days of treatment), among a long list of medications. Barbiturates and benzodiazepines can also trigger acute porphyria.
- Position and compression: If the weakness is triggered by a position that can result in nerve compression, especially if the compression is minimal, this suggests hereditary neuropathy with liability to pressure palsies (HNPP).

2. **Duration of weakness:** Weakness lasts for a few hours in patients with hyperkalemic PP, whereas patients with hypokalemic PP can have weakness for several hours or even days. Patients with MG can have weakness for several hours that extends to days or weeks. Patients with HNPP can have variable duration of the weakness, depending on the severity of the nerve compression. Patients with relapsing forms of chronic inflammatory demyelinating polyneuropathy (CIDP) can have weakness lasting for weeks or months.

3. **Distribution of weakness:** HNPP is suspected if the weakness is consistent within the territories of named peripheral nerves (e.g., foot drop due to peroneal nerve palsy or wrist drop due to radial nerve palsy). Primary weakness in the thighs and calves is seen in patients with hyperkalemic PP, although they can have generalized weakness. Patients with hypokalemic PP usually have generalized weakness, but facial and respiratory muscle weakness is rare in PPs. Conversely, facial and respiratory weakness as well as weakness of extraocular muscles (diplopia and ptosis) are suggestive of MG. Patients with acute intermittent porphyria can have generalized weakness, including bulbar and extraocular muscles, mimicking Guillain-Barré syndrome (GBS).

4. **Other manifestations:**
   - If the patient has evidence of myotonia or paramyotonia, this is suggestive of hyperkalemic PP. Myoglobinuria and muscle edema during weakness episodes suggest rhabdomyolysis. They can be seen in metabolic myopathies as well as in other myopathies that can present with recurrent rhabdomyolysis, such as ryanodinopathies and muscular dystrophies.
   - Family history of episodic weakness can be seen in several diseases such as the PP, metabolic myopathies, acute porphyria, and HNPP. The most common form of MG is acquired, so family history would suggest a congenital myasthenic syndrome.
   - Acute abdominal pain during weakness episodes can be seen in acute intermittent porphyria, although some patients with metabolic myopathies can also have abdominal pain associated with weakness and hemoglobinuria.

5. **Symptoms between attacks:** Patients with PP are usually asymptomatic between attacks, although patients with hyperkalemic PP can have myotonia or paramyotonia without weakness. With disease progression, patients with PP can develop chronic fixed weakness. Patients with MG can be asymptomatic between episodes or complain of generalized fatigue without focal weakness or episodic dysarthria, dyspnea, chewing, or swallowing problems. Patients with metabolic myopathies or recurrent rhabdomyolysis are usually asymptomatic between attacks.

6. **Other findings on the examination:**
   - Reflexes: Besides the distribution of weakness described earlier, the pattern of reflexes can differ by etiology. Reduced reflexes can be seen in patients with CIDP, hypokalemic PP (primary or secondary) during the attacks, and hypermagnesemia, and during attacks of acute intermittent porphyria. Patients with MG have normal reflexes during and in between attacks. Patients with HNPP can have normal or reduced reflexes, with the latter occurring if they also have a generalized polyneuropathy.
   - Sensory changes: Numbness following a focal peripheral nerve distribution suggests HNPP. Numbness in a glove/stocking distribution, like that observed in polyneuropathy, can be seen in relapsing CIDP, as well as in some patients with HNPP and in acute porphyria. The sensory examination is normal in the PPs, metabolic myopathies, and MG.
   - Myotonia or paramyotonia: These symptoms can be found in patients with hyperkalemic PP. They can be elicited by tapping (e.g., thenar eminence, extensor muscles of the forearm) or by action (e.g., eyelid myotonia or grip myotonia).

Exercise Intolerance

Exercise intolerance includes the development of cramps, contractures, myalgia, and hemoglobinuria during exercise, as well as extreme fatigue with exercise not necessarily associated with objective weakness.

- Cramps, myalgia, and hemoglobinuria that develop after a brief episode of intense exercise suggest a glycogen storage disease. If the symptoms improve with sustained submaximal effort ("second wind"), this is very suggestive of McArdle's disease, the most common form of glycogen storage disease.
- Cramps and myalgia with or without hemoglobinuria, when triggered by low-intensity sustained exercise, suggest a fatty acid oxidation disease.
- Some patients with MG complain of generalized fatigue after sustained exercise, and they might have secondary myalgia due to muscle fatigue. These patients, however, do not have cramps, abdominal pain, or myoglobinuria.
- Some patients with mitochondrial myopathies describe exercise intolerance with fatigue and myalgia.

INVESTIGATIONS

Acute Setting

- Potassium (K^+) levels: Both hypokalemia and hyperkalemia are known to cause of episodic weakness. These imbalances are often secondary to systemic disease such as hyperthyroidism, acute tubular necrosis, or hyperaldosteronism, or use of medications (Table 5.2). Therefore, thyroid-stimulating hormone, serum sodium, chloride, anion gap, and creatinine tests should be obtained to look for secondary causes.
- Calcium and magnesium levels: Alterations in calcium and magnesium levels can trigger muscle weakness.
- Creatine kinase (CK) levels: These can be moderately elevated in the acute phase of the periodic paralyses, and highly elevated in acute episodes of weakness or myalgia in the metabolic myopathies, particularly during an episode of rhabdomyolysis.

TABLE 5.2 Secondary Causes of Hypokalemia and Hyperkalemia

Hypokalemia	Hyperkalemia
Thyrotoxicosis	Hypoaldosteronism
Hyperaldosteronism	Addison's disease
Chronic diuretic medications	Rhabdomyolysis
Renal tubular acidosis	Potassium-sparing diuretic medications
Bartter's syndrome	Potassium supplementation
Amphotericin B toxicity	Chronic renal failure

CK should be normal in MG, HNPP, CIDP, and acute intermittent porphyria.

- Electrocardiography (EKG): Performing an EKG is fundamental in patients with hypokalemia or hyperkalemia because of the risk of arrhythmia. Patients with Anderson-Tawil syndrome can have long QT and other arrhythmias between attacks.
- Respiratory function tests: Reduced forced vital capacity (FVC) and inspiratory pressure may be associated with MG or acute intermittent porphyria with bulbar weakness.
- Lactate: The lactate level can be elevated in mitochondrial myopathies.

Electrodiagnostic Studies

- Electromyography (EMG): EMG can show fibrillations and positive sharps in acute episodes of PPs as well as rhabdomyolysis. Patients with hyperkalemic PP can also have myotonic discharges. In between attacks, myopathic units might be seen in metabolic and mitochondrial myopathies, although the EMG is often normal in these diseases. Patients with CIDP and HNPP can also have acute and/or chronic neurogenic changes.
- Nerve conduction studies (NCS): Compound motor action potentials (CMAPs) are reduced in patients with PPs during the weakness attacks, but are normal between episodes. NCS can show evidence of a demyelinating neuropathy in patients with HNPP or CIDP, and evidence of focal neuropathies in HNPP. An axonal neuropathy can be seen in acute intermittent porphyria. Routine NCS will be normal in MG and metabolic myopathies.
- Single fiber EMG (SFEMG): This test will show increased jitter and blocking in patients with MG, with very high sensitivity (more than 90%), especially if a weak muscle is tested. However, SFEMG is not specific for NMJ disorders, and increased jitter can be seen in patients with chronic myopathies, motor neuron disease, or acute rhabdomyolysis, and in the acute setting in PPs.
- Repetitive nerve stimulation (RNS): The typical test done at 3 Hz can show a decrement of more than 10% in patients with MG, with a sensitivity of approximately 70% for generalized disease. Patients with PPs can have normal RNS but could also have some decrement of CMAPs. Patients with myopathies, HNPP, and acute porphyria or CIDP have normal RNS studies.
- Short exercise test: This is done by recording the CMAP at baseline, and then every 10 seconds following 5 to 10 seconds of isometric contractions, for 1 minute. If there is any decrement, CMAP recording continues until it goes back to baseline. This test is usually normal in the PPs, but there can be transient increase in the CMAPs during an acute attack. CMAP decrement can be seen in

patients with MG. Patients with myopathies, HNPP, porphyria, or CIDP have normal short exercise test.

- Long exercise test: This is done by recording a baseline CMAP first, followed by muscle contraction for 3 to 5 minutes, with a few seconds of rest every 15 seconds. The CMAPs are recorded after 5 minutes of exercise and then every 1 to 2 minutes for 40 to 60 minutes. Patients with PPs show stable or slightly increased CMAP amplitude immediately after exercise, with progressive decline that peaks approximately after 30 minutes. Patients with MG can have a CMAP decrement after exercise, which may then recover with rest. This test is normal in other myopathies, HNPP, CIDP, and porphyria.

Forearm Exercise Test

The forearm exercise test has high sensitivity and specificity for glycogen storage disease. The test is performed after at least 15 minutes of rest. A catheter is inserted into a vein in the antecubital fossa, and lactate, pyruvate, and ammonia measurements are obtained at baseline. The patient is asked to do either intermittent contraction or persistent isometric contraction, and blood samples are repeated after the exercise. Patients with glycogen storage diseases have no rise in lactate level after exercise but do show increased ammonia levels. The nonischemic test is now preferred due to risk of compartment syndrome with the ischemic test.

Specific Workup

Acylcartinine profile is the most sensitive test for fatty acid oxidation disorders, and the yield can be increased by testing in the morning, ideally with the patient fasting. Urine porphobilinogens are abnormal in acute intermittent porphyria, with increased uroporphyrin and aminolevulinic acid levels being noted.

Muscle Biopsy

Muscle biopsy is rarely needed in patients with episodic weakness.

- Rimmed vacuoles can be seen in patients with PPs.
- Patients with glycogen storage disorders can have glycogen deposits seen with PAS staining, and myophosphorylase staining is reduced or absent in McArdle's disease.
- Patients with fatty acid oxidation disorders can have increased lipid deposits seen on oil red stains.
- Ragged red fibers can be found in patients with mitochondrial myopathies.
- Central cores can be seen in central-core disease or other ryanodine-related disorders.
- A dystrophic pattern can be seen in recurrent rhabdomyolysis associated with muscular dystrophies.

Genetic Testing

Specific genetic testing is available for the channelopathies that cause PP, as well as for the most common metabolic myopathies. Patients with suspected HNPP and acute intermittent porphyria can also undergo genetic testing.

Table 5.3 summarizes the findings on these tests according to the underlying cause of episodic weakness.

DIFFERENTIAL DIAGNOSIS

The differential diagnosis of episodic weakness depends on the clinical features obtained from the history and physical examination, especially the duration of weakness, triggering factors, and associated symptoms. The causes of episodic weakness can be broadly categorized by anatomic localization: nerve, NMJ, or muscle, with the additional category of endocrinologic or metabolic derangements.

1. **Nerve:** Think of a nerve localization if the patient has both sensory and motor manifestations (although these conditions may be motor predominant), the weakness follows a myotomal distribution or the distribution of specific peripheral nerves, or other features support a peripheral neuropathy (such as reduced or absent reflexes).
   - Patients with relapsing forms of immune-mediated neuropathies, such as CIDP, may present with episodes of weakness, which are often responsive to immunotherapy.
   - Patients with HNPP may develop focal neurologic deficits within the distribution of specific peripheral nerves at common sites of compression (e.g., median nerve at the wrist, ulnar nerve at the elbow, fibular nerve at the knee, or brachial plexus). These deficits usually improve over the course of days to weeks.
   - Patients with acute intermittent porphyria often present with acute generalized weakness, mimicking GBS, but with additional prominent autonomic involvement (with abdominal pain being particularly common) and psychiatric manifestations (anxiety, confusion, psychosis).
2. **Neuromuscular junction (NMJ):** Think of a NMJ localization especially in a patient with a pure motor syndrome, with extraocular manifestations (ptosis, diplopia), and symptoms that fluctuate with activity or diurnally.
   - MG classically produces fluctuating and fatigable weakness involving extraocular, bulbar, limb, or respiratory muscles. The weakness may worsen with prolonged activity and improve with rest or sleep. In addition, weakness is responsive to immunotherapy and/or acetylcholinesterase inhibitors.

TABLE 5.3 Laboratory Findings in Different Disease Causing Episodic Weakness and/or Exercise Intolerance

	Hypokalemic PP	Hyperkalemic PP	MG	Glycogen storage disorders	Fatty acid oxidation disorders	Recurrent rhabdomyolysis (not metabolic myopathy)	HNPP	Acute intermittent porphyria
Serum K^+	Reduced during attack, normal between attacks	Elevated or normal during attack, normal between	Normal	Normal; can be elevated during rhabdomyolysis	Normal; can be elevated during rhabdomyolysis	Can be elevated in acute setting	Normal	Normal
CK	Elevated during attacks, normal in between	Elevated during attacks, normal in between	Normal	Highly elevated during and between attacks	Highly elevated during attacks, normal or elevated in between	Extremely elevated during attacks, normal or elevated in between attacks	Normal	Normal
EKG	Can be abnormal during attack due to low K^+; abnormal between attacks suggests Andersen-Tawil syndrome	Can be abnormal during attack due to K^+; abnormal between attacks suggests Andersen-Tawil syndrome	Normal	Normal	Normal	Normal	Normal	Normal. Can have arrhythmia is severe autonomic dysfunction

(continued)

116

TABLE 5.3 Laboratory Findings in Different Disease Causing Episodic Weakness and/or Exercise Intolerance (continued)

	Hypokalemic PP	Hyperkalemic PP	MG	Glycogen storage disorders	Fatty acid oxidation disorders	Recurrent rhabdomyolysis (not metabolic myopathy)	HNPP	Acute intermittent porphyria
EMG	During attack insertional activity can be increased; between attacks normal or myopathic	Can have myotonic discharges; during attacks with fibrillations; between attacks normal or myopathic MUAPs	Normal. Rarely myopathic in patients with long-standing fixed weakness.	Usually normal; can show electrical silence during a contracture	Can show fibrillations in acute episode; between episodes can be normal or myopathic	Can show fibrillations in acute episode; between episodes can be normal or myopathic	Can be normal or have acute and chronic neurogenic changes in focal nerve territories	Can be normal or acute/chronic neurogenic changes
NCS	CMAPs can be reduced during acute attack; otherwise normal	CMAPs can be reduced during acute attack; otherwise normal	Normal	Normal	Normal	Normal	Evidence of focal neuropathies and/or demyelinating polyneuropathy	Axonal sensory and motor changes
RNS	Normal or decrement	Normal or decrement	Decrement > 10%	Normal	Normal	Normal	Normal	Normal
SFEMG	Can have increased jitter and blocking during acute attack; normal between attacks	Can have increased jitter and blocking during acute attack; normal between attacks	Abnormal, increased jitter, blocks	Normal, but can be abnormal in acute setting if there is rhabdomyolysis	Normal, but can be abnormal in acute setting if there is rhabdomyolysis	Can have increased jitter and blocks during acute attack; normal between attacks	Normal	Normal

(continued)

TABLE 5.3 Laboratory Findings in Different Disease Causing Episodic Weakness and/or Exercise Intolerance (*continued*)

	Hypokalemic PP	Hyperkalemic PP	MG	Glycogen storage disorders	Fatty acid oxidation disorders	Recurrent rhabdomyolysis (not metabolic myopathy)	HNPP	Acute intermittent porphyria
Long exercise test	Initial increase in CMAP, followed by progressive drop (~50%) after 20–40 minutes	Initial increase in CMAP, followed by progressive drop (~50%) after 20–40 minutes	Can have decrement in CMAP	Progressive decrement in CMAP after ~ 30 minutes	Normal	Normal	Normal	Normal
Short exercise test	Normal or increase in CMAP amplitude during attack	Normal or increase in CMAP amplitude during attack	Can have decrement in CMAP	Normal	Normal	Normal	Normal	Normal
Forearm test	Normal	Normal	Normal	Normal rise in ammonia, but no rise in lactic acid	Normal	Normal	Normal	Normal

CK, creatine kinase; CMAP, compound motor action potential; EKG, electrocardiography; EMG, electromyography; HNPP, hereditary neuropathy with liability to pressure palsies; MG, myasthenia gravis; MUAP, motor unit action potential; NCS, nerve conduction study; PP, periodic paralysis; RNS, repetitive nerve stimulation; SFEMG, single fiber EMG.

3. **Muscle:**
   - The channelopathies are a group of autosomal dominant genetically determined diseases, involving individual ion channels in muscle, which can lead to PP. The weakness can be diffuse or more focal, and can last from hours to days. The most common channelopathies are those that cause hypokalemic PP (due to mutations in the voltage-gated calcium channel [CACNA1S], or voltage-gated sodium channel [SCN4A]), or hyperkalemic PP (due to mutations in the voltage-gated sodium channel [SCN4A]). The presence of myotonic discharges on EMG can help point the diagnosis toward hyperkalemic PP.
   - The metabolic myopathies are a heterogeneous group of genetically determined muscle diseases (most are autosomal recessive) that can be divided into glycogen storage diseases (if due to abnormalities in the metabolism of glucose), lipid storage myopathies (if due to fatty acid oxidation defects), or mitochondrial myopathies. They may present with some element of exercise intolerance, contractures, and myoglobinuria.
   - Other inherited forms of myopathy may also present with rhabdomyolysis and, therefore, with episodic weakness, including those from ryanodine receptor mutations and some forms of muscular dystrophy (e.g., dystrophinopathy, dysferlinopathy, fukutin-related protein [FKRP] mutations, among others).
4. **Endocrinologic and other metabolic derangements that can produce episodic weakness:**
   - Thyrotoxic PP is a rare complication of hyperthyroidism, and can mimic the features of hypokalemic PP. Thus, thyroid function should be checked in all patients in whom PP is suspected.
   - Secondary causes of hypokalemia or hyperkalemia may cause episodic weakness at the time of the metabolic derangement. Table 5.2 lists many secondary causes of hypokalemia and hyperkalemia. Hypophosphatemia can lead to generalized weakness, sometimes associated with ileus and myoglobinuria. Hypermagnesemia can cause weakness and in severe cases is associated with flaccid quadriplegia, absent deep tendon reflexes, and respiratory failure. Derangements in calcium homeostasis can also lead to generalized weakness.

TREATMENT

- The details of treatment strategies and dosing are beyond the scope of this chapter, but the following summary provides general information about the treatment options for many of the diseases that may cause episodic weakness. This section is organized similarly to the preceding differential diagnosis section.

Nerve

- Treatment of CIDP involves immunotherapy, with first-line agents including corticosteroids (oral or intravenous), intravenous immunoglobulin, or plasma exchange.
- There is no specific treatment for HNPP apart from avoiding activities or positions that result in compression on nerves (e.g., avoiding elbow leaning or leg crossing).
- Acute intermittent porphyria attacks are treated with supportive therapy, in addition to intravenous heme (hemin). Carbohydrate loading may be used in milder cases, or while awaiting the availability of hemin.

Neuromuscular Junction

- The treatment of MG is complex, and depends on the presence of purely ocular or generalized features, disease severity, and response to first-line agents. For symptomatic management, oral pyridostigmine is first-line therapy, and may be sufficient in very mild purely ocular cases. Chronic management of many ocular cases and generalized MG involves immunotherapy, with corticosteroids being the first-line agents. Steroid-sparing agents are used in more severe cases, or when steroids cannot be adequately tapered; they include methotrexate, mycophenolate mofetil, and azathioprine. For acute exacerbations of MG, particularly involving bulbar or respiratory weakness, plasma exchange or intravenous immunoglobulins are the treatment of choice. Supportive care and close clinical monitoring are critical in these cases.

Muscle

- The treatment of PP due to channelopathies can be divided into acute treatment and preventive treatment. An acute paralytic attack of hypokalemic PP can be treated conservatively (monitoring), or in cases with a documented low-serum potassium, careful administration of oral potassium chloride (with cardiac monitoring) can be considered. Preventive management of hypokalemic PP includes a low-carbohydrate diet and avoidance of intense physical exercise. In addition, regular oral potassium supplementation and potassium-sparing diuretics can be used to maintain serum potassium levels. Carbonic anhydrase inhibitors, such as acetazolamide, are also used prophylactically to reduce attack frequency.
- With hyperkalemic PP, acute attacks are often brief, and may be treated with exercise or oral carbohydrate intake. Measures to reduce serum potassium can be used in more prolonged attacks, such as diuretics or inhaled beta-agonists. For prevention of attacks, patients can avoid foods rich in potassium. Carbonic

anhydrase inhibitors can also be utilized as prophylactic management to avoid paralytic attacks.
- Management of the metabolic myopathies in general involves avoidance of activities that induce myoglobinuria.
- For the glycogen storage diseases, patients may attempt to avoid high-intensity exercise, or gradually increase the intensity of exercise. Other potential treatments are sometimes attempted (such as creatine monohydrate, or carbohydrate loading before exercise), but these have not been unequivocally demonstrated to be beneficial in clinical trials. In some patients with McArdle's disease, there is a secondary vitamin B_6 deficiency, and so supplementation may be considered, but no trials exist in this regard. Caution should be used with vitamin B_6 supplementation, as higher doses can cause a sensory ganglionopathy.
- For the fatty acid oxidation diseases, a high-carbohydrate, low-fat diet is generally recommended, as is avoidance of fasting. In patients with a low L-carnitine level, this may be supplemented. A small retrospective study showed that triheptanoin may improve exercise capacity.
- No specific disease-modifying therapy exists currently for mitochondrial myopathies. However, some experts recommend a cocktail that may include coenzyme Q10, riboflavin, vitamin E, alpha-lipoic acid, and creatine monohydrate.
- If a patient develops rhabdomyolysis with myoglobinuria, regardless of cause, the management should include intravenous hydration, monitoring, and correction of electrolyte abnormalities (including cardiac monitoring if there is evidence of hyperkalemia), and careful monitoring of renal function to identify renal failure early. Patients who develop renal impairment should have a nephrology consultation and may need dialysis in severe cases.

Endocrinologic and Metabolic

- Treatment is generally directed at correcting the metabolic derangement, as well as investigating and treating the underlying cause. In cases of thyrotoxic PP, establishment of a euthyroid state should eliminate paralytic attacks.

SUGGESTED READING

Gilhus NE. Myasthenia gravis. *N Engl J Med.* 2016;375(26):2570–2581.

Kung AW. Neuromuscular complications of thyrotoxicosis. *Clin Endocrinol (Oxf).* 2007;67:645–650.

Olpin SE, Murphy E, Kirk RJ, et al. The investigation and management of metabolic myopathies. *J Clin Pathol.* 2015;68:410–417. doi:10.1136/jclinpath-2014-202808

Pischik E, Kauppinen R. An update of clinical management of acute intermittent porphyria. *Appl Clin Genet.* 2015;8:201–214. doi:10.2147/TACG.S48605

Platt D, Griggs R. Skeletal muscle channelopathies: new insights into the periodic paralyses and nondystrophic myotonias. *Curr Opin Neurol.* 2009;22(5):524–531.

Tarnopolsky MA. Metabolic myopathies. *Continuum (Minneap Minn).* 2016;22(6, Muscle and Neuromuscular Junction Disorders):1829–1851.

Venance SL, Cannon SC, Fialho D, et al. The primary periodic paralyses: diagnosis, pathogenesis and treatment. *Brain.* 2005;129(1):8–17.

6   Ocular and Bulbar Symptoms

Michael K. Hehir

Ocular and bulbar muscle dysfunction is observed in several neuromuscular disorders. The presence of weakness in these muscle groups is helpful in localizing a patient's symptoms within the peripheral nervous system and in narrowing the differential diagnosis to guide workup and management decisions. In neuromuscular disorders, ocular weakness may include eye movement abnormalities resulting in binocular diplopia, eyelid levator weakness resulting in ptosis, and orbicularis oculi weakness resulting in eye closure weakness. Bulbar dysfunction refers to oral and pharyngeal muscle weakness and results in the symptoms of dysphagia, dysarthria, and dysfunctional mastication.

This chapter discusses the symptoms and signs of ocular and bulbar muscle weakness in the context of disorders of the peripheral nervous system. It also discusses the development of a focused differential diagnosis of ocular and bulbar dysfunction based on history and physical exam findings and use of this focused differential diagnosis to guide evaluation and management decisions.

SYMPTOMS AND SIGNS

Localization within the nervous system is best accomplished by taking a detailed clinical history to generate an anatomic localization hypothesis. A detailed neurologic exam is performed to confirm or refute this hypothesis. This section provides potential anatomic localizations for ocular and bulbar dysfunction and discusses how a detailed history and clinical exam can be used to determine appropriate localization in a symptomatic patient.

Clinicians can take advantage of the concept of selective vulnerability of certain regions of the nervous system in neuromuscular disorders to guide anatomic localization. In addition, the constellation of symptoms outside the ocular and bulbar regions can assist clinicians in narrowing a differential diagnosis.

Peripheral Nerve

Generalized peripheral neuropathies are a rare cause of ocular and bulbar weakness. Isolated cranial nerve disorders are more common.

- Abnormalities with examination of deep tendon reflexes, sensory function, and gait ataxia suggest localization in the peripheral nervous system.
- Patients with isolated ocular findings that localize to a specific cranial nerve should be carefully assessed for other signs of brainstem dysfunction, cavernous sinus disease, and multiple cranial neuropathies.
- Acute-onset ocular weakness and bulbar dysfunction with associated sensory symptoms in limbs and gait ataxia are indicative of either pure Miller Fisher syndrome or generalized Guillain-Barré syndrome (GBS) with features of Miller Fisher syndrome.

Motor Neuron Disease

Disease of the motor neurons results in a pure motor syndrome. Bulbar muscle involvement is common. Ocular weakness is atypical and should prompt clinicians to consider alternative anatomic localization.

- Classical amyotrophic lateral sclerosis (ALS) is associated with a combination of upper and lower motor neuron findings in affected limbs. Pure lower motor neuron (progressive muscular atrophy [PMA]) and pure upper motor neuron (primary lateral sclerosis [PLS]) can also be associated with bulbar dysfunction. About one-third of patients with ALS will present with bulbar palsy at onset.
- ALS, PMA, and PLS are asymmetric. Symmetric findings should prompt clinicians to consider alternative etiologies.
- Both mild cognitive impairment and frontotemporal dementia can be associated with ALS.

Neuromuscular Junction

Patients with neuromuscular junction (NMJ) disorders have a pure motor syndrome. NMJ disorders can cause ocular weakness, bulbar weakness, or both.

- Generalized myasthenia gravis typically has an acute or subacute onset. It tends to involve neck flexion, shoulder abduction, hip flexion, hip abduction, and respiratory muscles, in addition to the ocular and bulbar muscles.
- Patients with myasthenia gravis typically have symptoms and signs of fatigable weakness. Muscle function declines with extended use and at times when the patient is tired. Provocative maneuvers can be used to evaluate this condition at the bedside.
- Lambert-Eaton myasthenic syndrome (LEMS) is a chronic disorder that tends to cause significant proximal lower extremity weakness out of proportion to weakness in other muscles.

- Botulism causes rapidly progressive weakness in a similar ana-tomic distribution to myasthenia gravis. Given the rapidity of onset, patients may not demonstrate fatigability or facilitation on exam.
- LEMS and botulism can be associated with autonomic dysfunc-tion due to preganglionic autonomic pathology.

Muscle

Myopathies can be associated with ocular weakness, bulbar weak-ness, or both. Some myopathies can have manifestations outside the peripheral nervous system that can be clues to diagnosis.

- Muscular dystrophies tend to have a chronic course. While de novo cases are possible, many patients have a history of affected family members.
- Muscular dystrophies also tend to have specific patterns of weak-ness due to muscle selective vulnerability (e.g., fascioscapulo-humeral muscular dystrophy [FSHD] causes asymmetric facial weakness, scapular winging, proximal lower extremity weakness, dorsiflexion weakness, and lower abdominal weakness).
- Patients with oculopharyngeal muscular dystrophy (OPMD) may have signs of mild to moderate proximal limb weakness in addi-tion to ptosis, dysphagia, and dysarthria.
- In addition to the classical pattern of weakness and myoto-nia, patients with myotonic dystrophy type 1 will exhibit many extra-muscular manifestations, including cataracts, cardiac arrhythmia, sleep apnea, and cognitive dysfunction.
- Mitochondrial myopathies causing progressive external ophthal-moplegia (PEO) tend to occur in younger patients. Kearns-Sayre syndrome may be associated with cardiac abnormality and cer-ebellar dysfunction. Sensory ataxic neuropathy, dysarthria, and ophthalmoparesis (SANDO) are associated with peripheral neu-ropathy and ataxia.

Ocular Muscle Dysfunction

Orbital muscle, eyelid levator, and orbicularis oculi muscle dysfunc-tion result in a combination of symptoms including diplopia, ptosis, and difficult eye closure. Ocular muscle dysfunction can result from the following causes:

- Supranuclear lesions
- Brainstem disease (e.g., intranuclear ophthalmoplegia in multiple sclerosis)
- Cranial nerve dysfunction (e.g., sixth cranial nerve palsy)
- NMJ dysfunction (e.g., myasthenia gravis)

- Ocular muscle weakness (e.g., OPMD)
- Orbital muscle restriction (e.g., orbital mass lesion)
- Ocular refractive error (e.g., astigmatism)

Diplopia

Diplopia is the symptom of double vision. It can be caused by either a refractive error or dysconjugate gaze. In both cases, each eye receives a single target image in a slightly different region of macula. The target is transmitted to the visual cortex as a double image.

Non-neuromuscular Diplopia

- Monocular diplopia—that is, double image perceived with only one eye open—is typically the result of a refractive error. In many instances, monocular diplopia can be corrected at the bedside by asking the patient to look through a pinhole.
- Orbital muscle restriction due to an orbital mass lesion or ocular muscle fibrosis can result in mechanical dysconjugate gaze. A forced duction test can be performed in an ophthalmology clinic; inability to passively move the eye beyond the maximal point achieved with voluntary movement with special forceps indicates globe restriction. Patients will often experience double vision in a particular direction of gaze. They may also have concurrent proptosis or pain.
- Patients should be questioned about a history of long-standing esotropia or exotropia, which can mimic a neuromuscular disorder or cranial neuropathy.

Neuromuscular Diplopia

Diplopia due to neuromuscular weakness is always binocular and the result of dysconjugate gaze. Patients may experience mild diplopia as blurry vision. Diplopia related to dysconjugate gaze always improves when covering either eye. Patients may describe:

- Persistent double vision in all directions of gaze that improves when either eye is covered.
- Fluctuating diplopia that is worse with eye strain (e.g., prolonged driving) or when the patient is fatigued (e.g., end of day or after poor sleep). This finding is suggestive of myasthenia gravis.
- Light sensitivity, which may be experienced as a form of mild diplopia in myasthenia gravis.
- Neuromuscular disorders (e.g., OPMD, PEO) that are associated with dysconjugate gaze or restricted eye movements without the symptom of diplopia.

Ptosis

Eyelid levator function is controlled by the combined function of the levator palpebrae superioris, Müller's muscle, and the frontalis muscle. Dysfunction in these muscles results in unintended eyelid closure. Similarly to diplopia, time course, associated symptoms and signs, and a thorough exam can help determine etiology.

Central Nervous System–Associated Ptosis

- Supranuclear lesions can produce unilateral ptosis, bilateral ptosis, or eyelid opening apraxia.
- Brainstem lesions affecting the nucleus of cranial nerve III can result in unilateral ptosis. These lesions are accompanied by other symptoms and signs of cortical or brainstem dysfunction.

Autonomic Nervous System–Associated Ptosis

Parasympathetic dysfunction:

- Lesions affecting the parasympathetic fibers in cranial nerve III can result in a combination of ptosis and mydriasis due to denervation of the levator palpebrae superioris muscle and unopposed sympathetic input to the pupillary sphincter.
- Isolated parasympathetic cranial nerve III lesions are typically the result of compression because the parasympathetic fibers are somatotopically located in the periphery of the nerve.
- In the acute setting, isolated ptosis and mydriasis (colloquially a "blown pupil") is a neurologic emergency. Potential etiologies include intracranial aneurysm, cavernous sinus pathology, mass lesion, and rising intracranial pressure.

Sympathetic Dysfunction

- Horner syndrome is due to lesions of the oculosympathetic pathway. It results in the clinical findings of ptosis (Müller's muscle denervation), miosis (unopposed parasympathetic input to pupillary muscles), and facial anhydrosis (if sympathetic innervations of the face are involved).
- Provocative testing in the ophthalmology clinic with cocaine eye drops can confirm the presence of Horner syndrome.
- Horner syndrome can result from lesions anywhere along the pathway of oculosympathetic fibers, which originate in the hypothalamus and traverse the brainstem, lateral cervical spinal cord, sympathetic trunk, carotid artery, skull base, cavernous sinus, and orbit.

Neuromuscular Ptosis

Neuromuscular Junction:

- Ptosis due to NMJ lesions often occurs in an acute or subacute time frame.
- Fluctuating ptosis is often observed in myasthenia gravis and often noticed by the patient at the end of the day, when fatigued, and with eye strain.

- NMJ-induced ptosis is often associated with orbicularis oculi weakness and eye closure dysfunction.

Muscle

- Ptosis due to myopathies tends to develop chronically and is often associated with weakness of facial muscles, bulbar muscles, and limb muscles.
- OPMD and mitochondrial myopathies can also be associated with eye movement abnormalities. Either due to chronicity of onset or symmetric involvement of ocular muscles, many of these patients do not experience diplopia.
- Myotonic dystrophy type 1 does not typically cause concurrent ocular muscle weakness.

Physical Exam in Patient With Diplopia and/or Ptosis

A detailed physical exam in the patient presenting with diplopia and/or ptosis due to possible neuromuscular disorder can help to provide evidence for anatomic localization and etiology. All patients presenting with possible neuromuscular induced ptosis and diplopia should be evaluated for concurrent bulbar and respiratory muscle weakness. Following are clinical pearls that may help with diagnosis.

Diplopia

- Each eye should be covered independently to evaluate whether the double image is monocular or binocular. Monocular double vision is indicative of a refractive error; a pinhole exam can help confirm this diagnosis at the bedside.
- Visual acuity should be assessed in all patients presenting for ocular symptoms.
- A red glass or Maddox rod can be utilized to localize eye muscle weakness. The image perceived as more lateral by the patient is attributable to the weak eye.
- A forced duction test with local anesthesia can be performed in an ophthalmology clinic to evaluate for globe restriction.
- Patients should be asked to hold their gaze in the horizontal and vertical plane for 1 to 2 minutes. Development of diplopia and/or dysconjugate gaze is supportive of NMJ pathology.
- Eye movement abnormalities without reported diplopia may be indicative of chronic myopathy (e.g., OPMD, PEO).
- Careful evaluation of sensory function, deep tendon reflexes, gait, and limb function should be performed to assess for concurrent signs of peripheral nerve, NMJ, and/or muscle dysfunction.

Ptosis

- Evaluating an older photo of the patient (e.g., driver's license) can help to establish duration of symptoms in cases where onset is unclear.
- Multiple tests for fluctuating ptosis indicative of NMJ disease should be performed:
  - Sustained upward gaze by the patient for 1 to 2 minutes should be assessed. Ptosis in myasthenia gravis will become more apparent with sustained gaze.
  - The "curtain sign" is demonstrated when the examiner lifts the more affected eyelid and this action results in worsened ptosis on the contralateral, less affected side.
  - Cogan's lid twitch can also be observed. After a patient has directed the eyes downward for 20 to 30 seconds, the patient is asked to look up. Affected eyelids will twitch before settling in baseline position with ptosis.
  - An ice test can also be performed in the office. An ice bag is applied to the eyelids for 2 to 5 minutes. In myasthenia gravis, ptosis will partially or fully resolve because cold temperature slows the chemical reaction that breaks down acetylcholine.
  - Although often unnecessary, an edrophonium test can be performed in the clinic. Administration of this short-acting acetylcholinesterase inhibitor should resolve ptosis within about 30 seconds of administration. The test must be performed with cardiac monitoring and with rescue atropine available should the patient develop bradycardia and hypotension.
- Eye closure should be evaluated. Patients with NMJ, muscle, and peripheral nerve lesions can develop facial weakness.
- Careful evaluation of other cranial nerve function, deep tendon reflexes, gait, and limb function should be performed to assess for concurrent signs of peripheral nerve, NMJ, and/or muscle dysfunction.

Bulbar Muscle Dysfunction

Bulbar muscle dysfunction is the result of oral and pharyngeal muscle weakness. It results in the combination of dysphagia, dysarthria, and mastication dysfunction. Bulbar dysfunction can result from the following causes:

- Supranuclear lesions (e.g., stroke)
- Brainstem disease (e.g., stroke, demyelination)
- Cranial nerve dysfunction
- Peripheral nerve disease (e.g., GBS)

- NMJ dysfunction (e.g., myasthenia gravis)
- Primary muscle weakness

Dysphagia

Oral and pharyngeal muscle dysfunction can impair the act of swallowing. Patients with oral and pharyngeal dysphagia experience a combination of symptoms:

- Coughing may occur with eating or drinking due to aspiration. Difficulty with thin liquids and mixed consistencies (e.g., soup) is often the first sign of neuromuscular dysphagia.
- Escape of fluid from nose with drinking is indicative of soft palate weakness. This symptom raises concern for myasthenia gravis.
- Increasing duration of meals can be indicative of both dysphagia and difficulty with mastication.
- Severe inability to swallow secretions can result in sialorrhea. This symptom can cause significant morbidity in the late stages of neuromuscular diseases such as ALS.
- Weight loss may occur due to inadequate caloric intake.
- Recurrent aspiration pneumonias may be reported.

Esophageal dysphagia is often experienced as sensation that food is stuck in the neck or chest after transit through the oral pharynx. Esophageal dysfunction is atypical of neuromuscular disorders. If suspected, patients should be referred to a gastroenterologist for evaluation.

Dysarthria

Neuromuscular disorders affecting the bulbar musculature are typically associated with flaccid dysarthria due to lower motor neuron, NMJ, or muscle dysfunction. The exception is ALS. Classical ALS results in a mixed upper and lower motor neuron–induced dysarthria with both spastic and flaccid components. Neuromuscular patients with dysarthria can experience a combination of the following symptoms:

- Hypophonia due to oropharyngeal dysfunction and/or respiratory muscle dysfunction.
- Nasal dysarthria with escape of air through the soft palate. This type of dysarthria is typical of myasthenia gravis.
- Guttural dysarthria, or difficulty pronouncing hard sounds (e.g., K and G), which can indicate pharyngeal dysfunction.
- Buccal dysarthria, or difficulty pronouncing M or W sounds, which can be indicative of orbicularis oris weakness. This can be associated with inability to drink from a straw, whistle, and smile.

- Mixed flaccid and spastic dysarthria, often described as a strained pattern of speech by patients and families.

Dysarthria can be a source of great morbidity for patients with neuromuscular disorders, as it impedes the essential human function of effective communication. In many patients, an early sign of dysarthria will be inability for others to understand speech over the telephone due to the lack of visual input for the listener.

History and Physical Exam
The clinical history of the patient presenting with dysphagia and dysarthria due to possible neuromuscular disorder can help to provide a hypothesis for anatomic localization and etiology. Following are clinical pearls that may help with diagnosis.

History
- Time course:
  - Acute to subacute:
    - Peripheral nerve disease (e.g., GBS)
    - Bulbar-onset motor neuron disease (e.g., ALS)
    - NMJ (myasthenia gravis, botulism)
  - Chronic:
    - Motor neuron disease limb onset (e.g., ALS)
    - Muscular dystrophy (e.g., OPMD)
- Quality of dysphagia:
  - Coughing with swallowing liquids, mixed consistencies, and oral secretions is indicative of oral pharyngeal weakness.
  - Loss of fluid from the nose is indicative of soft palate weakness observed in NMJ disease.
  - Symptoms of esophageal dysphagia are indicative of a non-neuromuscular etiology.
- Quality of dysarthria:
  - Nasal dysarthria is indicative of NMJ disease.
  - Strained speech is indicative of the mixed flaccid and spastic dysarthria of ALS.
  - Buccal dysarthria is indicative of facial weakness (e.g., FSHD)
  - Dysarthria that develops or worsens with prolonged periods of speaking or at the end of the day is suggestive of myasthenia gravis.

Physical Exam
- Dysphagia:
  - Patients should be observed for signs of aspiration of oral secretions. Patients may cough or clear the throat during the exam.

- A bedside clinical swallowing evaluation can be performed if the patient does not report aspiration of large volumes of oral contents. The patient is asked to drink 3 oz of water. If the individual coughs during or following this test, the patient may have signs of oropharyngeal dysphagia. The patient can be referred to a speech-language pathologist for additional testing.
- Dysarthria:
  - Examination of buccal, lingual, and guttural speech should be performed to help localize the area of dysfunction.
  - Asking the patient to hold a prolonged note can identify a spastic component to speech.
  - Fatigability of speech can be assessed by asking a patient to count out loud to the number 50 or 100. Development of progressive dysarthria during this exercise may indicate a NMJ disorder.
- Assess respiratory function:

  Many patients with neuromuscular disorders accompanied by bulbar muscle dysfunction are at risk to develop concurrent respiratory muscle dysfunction. Neuromuscular respiratory weakness is discussed in detail in another chapter of this text. At the bedside one can assess:
  - Ability to count out loud in a single breath.
  - Neck flexion strength in the supine position.
  - Strength of cough.
  - Some neuromuscular clinics also have the ability to check forced vital capacity, mean inspiratory pressure, and mean expiratory pressure.

DIFFERENTIAL DIAGNOSIS

Determining anatomic localization and duration of symptoms and signs is essential to narrow the differential diagnosis and guide the workup for the patient presenting with ocular and bulbar weakness. Table 6.1 presents a differential diagnosis for ocular and bulbar weakness based on symptoms and time course. The list can be prioritized further by including associated non-bulbar and ocular findings (e.g., limb hyperreflexia in ALS, ataxia in Miller Fisher variant of GBS).

Peripheral Nerve
GBS

- Facial nerve dysfunction occurs in up to 70% of patients with GBS. About 40% of patients experience bulbar dysfunction. Rare patients develop oculomotor dysfunction.
- The majority of patients with GBS present with the combination of proximal and distal lower extremity weakness first; facial involvement often occurs later in the course.

TABLE 6.1 Differential Diagnosis for Ocular and Bulbar Weakness

Symptom/Sign	Time Course	
	Acute/Subacute	Chronic
Ptosis	Peripheral nerve: • Miller Fisher syndrome, GBS • NMJ: • Myasthenia gravis • Botulism	NMJ: • Myasthenia gravis • Lambert-Eaton syndrome • Congenital myasthenia Muscle: • OPMD • Mitochondrial myopathy • Myotonic dystrophy type 1 • Congenital myopathy
Diplopia due to dysconjugate gaze	Peripheral nerve: • Miller Fisher, GBS NMJ: • Myasthenia gravis • Botulism Muscle: • Orbital pseudotumor	NMJ: • Myasthenia gravis • Lambert-Eaton syndrome • Congenital myasthenia Muscle: • OPMD • Mitochondrial myopathy • Congenital myopathy • Graves ophthalmopathy
Bulbar dysfunction	Peripheral nerve: • GBS Motor nerve: • Bulbar-onset ALS NMJ: • Myasthenia gravis • Botulism • Tetanus Muscle: • Critical illness (myopathy/neuropathy)	Motor nerve: • ALS • PLS • Spinal muscular atrophy • Kennedy disease NMJ: • Myasthenia gravis Muscle: • OPMD • Mitochondrial myopathy • Myotonic dystrophy • FSHD • Limb-girdle muscular dystrophy • Inclusion body myositis • Dermatomyositis • Polymyositis

ALS, amyotrophic lateral sclerosis; FSHD, fascioscapulohumeral muscular dystrophy; GBS, Guillain-Barré syndrome; NMJ, neuromuscular junction; OPMD, oculopharyngeal muscular dystrophy; PLS, primary lateral sclerosis.

- Maximal weakness is observed within 4 weeks of symptom onset in GBS.
- Patients with the Miller Fisher variant of GBS have early involvement of oculomotor muscles. Miller Fisher syndrome is associated with anti-GQ1b antibodies and is characterized by the development of ophthalmoplegia, ataxia, and areflexia. Miller Fisher patients are at increased risk for Bickerstaff brainstem encephalitis.

Motor Nerve
ALS

- ALS typically causes a combination of asymmetric upper and lower motor neuron symptoms and signs. For example, mixed flaccid and spastic dysarthria and tongue atrophy/weakness with associated increased jaw-jerk reflex can be observed.
- Bulbar muscle dysfunction is inevitable as the disease progresses. About one-third of ALS patients have onset of weakness in the bulbar muscles (i.e., bulbar-onset ALS).
- Ocular muscle weakness and ptosis are uncommon symptoms of ALS.
- Asymmetric weakness, muscle atrophy, and fasciculations with associated hyperreflexia are typically observed in limb muscles.
- Muscle cramping is observed in many patients with ALS.
- Executive dysfunction, pseudobulbar affect, and frontotemporal dementia are associated with ALS. This can impact treatment strategies.

Neuromuscular Junction
Myasthenia Gravis

- Fluctuating ptosis and diplopia are observed in the majority of patients with myasthenia gravis (MG). About 30% will have pure ocular MG.
- A total of 70% to 80% of patients with MG have measurable antibodies directed against the acetylcholine receptor. Another 7% have antibodies directed against muscle receptor–specific kinase (MuSK).
- Nasal dysarthria and loss of fluid through the nose when drinking are observed with bulbar weakness in MG.
- Severe bulbar dysfunction, neck extensor, and early respiratory muscle weakness should raise concern for anti-MuSK MG.
- In rare cases, patients with bulbar weakness due to MG can develop respiratory crisis due to airway obstruction.
- Patients with bulbar symptoms in MG should be assessed for concurrent respiratory muscle weakness.

Botulism

- Progressive weakness results from permanent inhibition of acetylcholine release during infection with neurotoxin-secreting *Clostridium* species.
- Cranial nerve abnormalities occur first in most patients, followed by a descending paralysis.
- Pupillary abnormalities are observed in about 50% of patients.
- Nausea, vomiting, and diarrhea may precede onset of weakness.

LEMS

- Ocular and bulbar symptoms are rare in LEMS. Progressive limb weakness is more common.
- LEMS is associated with preganglionic voltage-gated calcium-channel antibodies.
- LEMS is classically categorized as a paraneoplastic syndrome and associated with small cell lung cancer. Idiopathic autoimmune versions are also observed.
- Cases of concurrent LEMS and MG are rarely reported.

Muscle
OPMD

- OPMD typically manifests with a combination of ptosis and dysphagia in the fifth or sixth decade of life. Earlier and later onset of OPMD is possible.
- Eye movement abnormalities occur less frequently. Patients with OPMD who exhibit eye movement restriction do not typically describe diplopia.
- Variable limb-girdle weakness occurs later in the disease course in most patients.

Mitochondrial Myopathies
PEO

- PEO typically presents in childhood or young adulthood with a combination of ptosis and ophthalmoplegia. Most patients do not report diplopia.
- Earlier age of onset is a distinguishing feature from OPMD.
- Patients can develop oropharyngeal and limb symptoms.
- PEO can develop into a PEO-plus syndrome. Patients must be monitored for cardiac conduction abnormalities, cardiomyopathy, renal disease, hepatic disease, diabetes mellitus, and hearing loss.

Kearns-Sayre Syndrome

- Patients with Kearns-Sayre syndrome (KSS) develop ophthalmoplegia and retinitis pigmentosa before age 20.

- These patients must also have at least one associated clinical feature, including heart block, cerebellar ataxia, or cerebrospinal fluid (CSF) protein elevation.
- Patients with KSS may also develop limb weakness, oropharyngeal weakness, cognitive dysfunction, growth hormone deficiency, and diabetes mellitus.

Congenital Myopathies

- Congenital myopathies are a heterogeneous group of muscle disorders that present in children. Recent advances in pathology and molecular genetics have allowed for improved genetic classification and understanding of the pathophysiology of these conditions.
- Ophthalmoparesis with or without ptosis is common in patients with centronuclear myopathies due to multiple genetic etiologies.
- Ryanodine receptor recessive mutations have been associated with both ocular and bulbar muscle weakness.
- Bulbar muscle dysfunction is prominent in nemaline myopathy, especially with NEB mutations, and centronuclear myopathy due to DMN2 mutations.

Myotonic Dystrophy Type 1 (DM1)

- DM1 is the most common muscular dystrophy.
- Bifacial weakness is a prominent typical feature of DM1. Adult patients have a typical pattern of frontal baldness, temporal wasting, and a narrow face.
- Patients also have weakness in finger flexors, intrinsic hand muscles, and dorsiflexors of feet.
- Many patients with DM1 describe dysarthria and dysphagia. Dysphagia may be in part related to esophageal dysmotility, in contrast to the dysphagia associated with other dystrophies.
- Extramuscular manifestations of DM1 include cataracts, sensorineural hearing loss, sleep disorders, cardiac arrhythmias, cognitive dysfunction, and a predisposition to certain malignancies.
- Congenital DM1 presents with a severe phenotype of generalized weakness in newborns or in utero. Facial muscle weakness can be associated with inability to feed and polyhydramnios.

Fascioscapulohumeral Muscular Dystrophy

- Patients with FSHD typically present with asymmetric facial weakness manifested as difficulty whistling, drinking from a straw, puckering lips, and producing facial expression. Eye closure can also be weak.
- Bulbar dysfunction causing dysarthria and dysphagia is rare.
- Patients develop a classical pattern of scapular fixation, combined with humeral, truncal, and lower extremity weakness. This

is manifested as winged scapula, flattened clavicles, pectoral atrophy, lower abdominal protuberance, lumbar lordosis, and steppage gait.

Limb-Girdle Muscular Dystrophy

- Limb-girdle muscular dystrophy (LGMD) is a heterogeneous group of muscular dystrophies that can present in children or adults.
- Most patients have a clinical phenotype that includes progressive proximal limb weakness.
- Facial muscle involvement is rare but described in certain subsets of patients.
- Advances in next-generation molecular genetic sequencing are improving genotypic diagnoses in LGMD.

Idiopathic Inflammatory Myopathies (Dermatomyositis/Polymyositis)

- Weakness of pharyngeal muscles may occur in advanced dermatomyositis (DM) and polymyositis (PM), resulting in dysphagia and dysarthria.
- Prior to developing bulbar symptoms, patients with DM and PM typically display a symmetrical pattern of proximal limb weakness.
- DM is often associated with classical skin findings (e.g., heliotropic rash, shawl sign).
- Adult DM is strongly associated with malignancy. Patients should be evaluated for concurrent malignancy.

Inclusion Body Myositis

- Dysphagia can occur in up to 50% of patients with sporadic inclusion body myositis (IBM).
- Patients may also experience bifacial weakness. In some instances, bifacial weakness precedes development of typical IBM limb weakness.
- IBM classically causes a combination of bilateral finger flexor and quadriceps weakness and atrophy.

Graves Ophthalmopathy

- Hyperthyroid-associated ophthalmopathy is characterized by the combination of proptosis and dysconjugate gaze, particularly with upward and lateral gaze.
- Ophthalmopathy is due to an inflammatory infiltrate of orbital contents and muscle hypertrophy.
- T_4/T_3 levels are typically elevated, with associated low levels of TSH.

- Thyroid ophthalmopathy can occur in the absence of TSH, T_4, and T_3 abnormalities. MRI can demonstrate muscle hypertrophy in these cases.
- Myasthenia gravis should be excluded in all patients presenting with possible Graves ophthalmopathy.

EVALUATION OF OCULAR AND BULBAR WEAKNESS IN NEUROMUSCULAR DISORDERS

The initial workup of the patient presenting with ocular and bulbar weakness is directed toward establishing the diagnosis of the causative neuromuscular disorder. It is important to separate causes of ocular and bulbar weakness that may be reversible with medical therapies from those conditions that are progressive and will be managed with supportive care. As described earlier, the list of differential diagnoses is established by taking a careful clinical history and performing a detailed neurologic exam. Confirmatory testing will involve a combination of laboratory tests, genetic testing, electromyography, nerve and muscle imaging, and tissue biopsies. The full diagnostic workup for each of the neuromuscular conditions associated with ocular and bulbar weakness is beyond the scope of this chapter.

Ptosis and Oculomotor Weakness

Multiple provocative bedside tests can be performed to establish disease of the NMJ as the source of ptosis (e.g., ice test). In patients with progressive neuromuscular disorders (e.g., OPMD, PEO), involvement of consultants in ophthalmology, neuro-ophthalmology, and oculoplastic surgery is necessary to establish the severity of eyelid levator and oculomotor weakness and to develop a treatment plan. Workup by these specialists will include measurement of formal visual fields, eye movements, and eyelid levator function. Refractive lens and surgical treatments will be guided by these evaluations.

Dysphagia

Formal evaluation of swallowing function includes referral to a speech-language pathologist (SLP), direct bedside examination of swallowing function, and videofluoroscopic swallowing evaluation (VSE) or fiberoptic endoscopic evaluation of swallowing (FEES). VSE and FEES allow the operator to better determine the weakest muscles in a patient's swallowing mechanism. This localizing information is useful due to muscle selective vulnerability in neuromuscular disorders. Bedside testing with varied food consistencies is essential to determine safe food consistencies in a particular patient so as to reduce the risk of aspiration. Successful swallowing modification strategies can also be demonstrated during this testing.

Dysarthria

Early involvement of an SLP experienced with neuromuscular disorders is essential to help manage the communication issues that arise with progressive dysarthria. A comprehensive SLP evaluation will measure the current level of deficit, predict future deficits, and assess the cognitive abilities of a patient. This information then guides the need for and choice of augmentative communication technologies.

TREATMENT STRATEGIES FOR OCULAR AND BULBAR NEUROMUSCULAR WEAKNESS

Treatment of potentially reversible neuromuscular causes of ocular and bulbar weakness (e.g., myasthenia gravis) should be directed toward addressing the disease itself with disease-modifying therapies. Short-term supportive care may be needed in these conditions while an effective treatment plan is established. Fortunately, the development of new genetic-based interventions is expanding the disease-modifying options for previously progressive genetic disorders (e.g., muscular dystrophies).

In patients with progressive neuromuscular causes of ocular and bulbar weakness (e.g., OPMD), a multidisciplinary long-term treatment strategy for ocular and bulbar weakness is needed to improve patient function.

Ptosis and Ocular Weakness

Ocular muscle weakness can result in the symptoms of diplopia and ptosis. In potentially reversible conditions such as myasthenia gravis, manipulation of vision may be necessary while developing an effective overall treatment plan. In patients with progressive neuromuscular disorders, vision and eyelid function may need to be chronically manipulated to improve function.

Diplopia

Treatment of diplopia is aimed at improving eye conjugacy. When it is not possible to correct dysconjugate gaze, visual occlusion may be necessary.

- Ocular occlusion with an eye patch or opaque plastic occluder placed over lenses should improve double vision in patients with diplopia due to dysconjugate gaze. Shifting vision occlusion should be considered temporary in conditions such as myasthenia gravis.
- Prism lenses can change the pathway of light to correct diplopia. This strategy is more successful in patients with fixed double vision rather than fluctuating double vision, like that observed in myasthenia gravis.
- Ocular muscle surgery and local botulinum injections are less helpful in neuromuscular disorders.

Ptosis

Patients with progressive neuromuscular ptosis may require surgical intervention or mechanical manipulation to improve vision.

- Mechanical eyelid crutches attached to corrective lens frames can be tried.
- Resection of the levator palpebrae aponeurosis can be trialed in patients with progressive ptosis (e.g., OPMD, PEO). This procedure may need to be repeated.
- Frontal suspension of the eyelids with skeletal muscle fascia or sling can also be considered in patients with progressive ptosis.
- Surgery is typically indicated when ptosis begins to interfere with vision.

Dysphagia

Dysphagia in progressive neuromuscular disorders can result in aspiration, choking, malnutrition, dehydration, weight loss, and sialorrhea. Treatment is directed toward developing a safe plan for nutritional intake and reducing symptoms such as sialorrhea. As the diseases progress, placement of a percutaneous endoscopic gastrostomy (PEG) may be needed to maintain nutritional status, if placement of such a device is consistent with the patient's goals of care. Although placement of a PEG improves enteral access, it does not eliminate the risk of oral content aspiration and possible resultant aspiration pneumonia.

In most progressive neuromuscular conditions, placement of a PEG is associated with increased survival, weight stabilization, and improved quality of life. Management of dysphagia may vary based on the specific neuromuscular condition. An experienced SLP can help guide the timing of PEG placement. It is recommended that PEG be placed by a proceduralist (e.g., gastroenterologist, surgeon, interventional radiologist) with experience treating patients with neuromuscular disorders.

Special Cases

Amyotrophic Lateral Sclerosis

Dysphagia is inevitable in ALS. Establishing a patient's goals of care early in the disease course is essential when developing an individualized treatment plan for dysphagia.

- Early strategies involve dietary modification and swallowing techniques. As the disease progresses, PEG placement is necessary to maintain adequate nutrition.
- Care should be provided in a comprehensive ALS multidisciplinary clinic that includes access to an SLP and nutritionist.
- Multiple studies have demonstrated improved weight stabilization and increased survival in patients with ALS who receive a PEG.

- PEG placement may also improve quality of life in patients with ALS.
- Placement of PEG does not preclude oral intake for pleasure.
- Involvement of a palliative care specialist is helpful in guiding the nutrition plan for patients with ALS.
- Use of dextromethorphan and quinidine, with the goal of treating pseudobulbar affect, improved bulbar function in a recent randomized controlled trial.

Timing of PEG

PEG placement should be considered when:

- Patient weight decreases below 10% of baseline weight.
- Respiratory muscle function is declining to a level that may increase the risks associated with the PEG placement procedure.
  - The American Academy of Neurology ALS guidelines from 2009 indicate that risk of PEG placement may be less if performed while forced vital capacity (FVC) is above 50% of the predicted value.
  - More recent data (2013) demonstrate safe PEG placement in experienced centers with FVC less than or equal to 30% of the predicted value. We have placed PEGs safely in our center with FVCs less than 30% of the predicted value.
  - Use of noninvasive positive-pressure ventilation (NIV) during the procedure may be needed when patients have low FVC.

Oculopharyngeal Muscular Dystrophy

While genetic-based disease-modifying strategies are under development for OPMD, current management of dysphagia is aimed toward improving nutritional intake. Management of dysphagia is unique, as both surgical and nonsurgical options have demonstrated efficacy.

- Cricopharyngeal myomotomy will alleviate symptoms of dysphagia. Dysphagia typically recurs over a period of years.
- Recurrent cricopharyngeal dilation procedures have also demonstrated safety and efficacy in OPMD.
- Protocols for local botulinum injection are under evaluation in OPMD.
- As the disease progresses to advanced stages, many patients will require placement of a PEG to maintain adequate nutritional intake.

Dysarthria and Loss of Ability to Communicate

Bulbar weakness in progressive neuromuscular disorders results in reduced ability of patients to communicate and interact with others.

Treatment is directed toward optimizing natural speech for as long as possible, followed by developing individualized augmented or alternative communication strategies. Involvement of an SLP who is knowledgeable about augmented communication early in the course of illness allows time to develop an effective communication plan for a patient.

- Augmented communication improves quality of life in patients with dysarthria due to progressive neuromuscular disorders. In patients with ALS, ability to interact via social media has also been shown to improve quality of life.
- Augmentative or alternative communication strategies range from low-tech options such as writing and communication boards to increasingly high-tech options such as tablet devices, computers, and eye-gaze systems. Brain–computer interface systems are also under development.
- A comprehensive augmented communication plan should include strategies for in-person communication, telephone communication, written/typed communication, and online communication.
- In conditions such as ALS and Duchenne muscular dystrophy, in which patients may have concurrent cognitive dysfunction, it is important to assess patient ability to use assistive technologies.
- Voice banking of a patient's actual voice is increasingly available if the need for a speech-generating device is anticipated in advance of developing significant dysarthria. This strategy allows a speech-generating device to project a recording of the patient's own voice instead of a generic computerized voice.

CONCLUSIONS

Ocular and bulbar weakness is a prominent feature of many neuromuscular disorders. Taking a detailed history and performing a comprehensive physical exam are essential to localize a patient's presenting symptoms to an anatomic site and thus narrow the range of possible diagnoses. Once a diagnosis is established, a multidisciplinary approach is essential to develop comprehensive plans to improve function for the patient with neuromuscular ocular and bulbar weakness.

SUGGESTED READING

Amato AA, Barohn RJ. Inclusion body myositis: old and new concepts. *J Neurol Neurosurg Psychiatry*. 2009;80:1186–1193.

Ball LJ, Fager S, Fried-Oken M. Augmentative and alternative communication for people with progressive neuromuscular disease. *Phys Med Rehabil Clin North Am*. 2012;23:689–699.

Brais B. Oculopharyngeal muscular dystrophy: a polyalanine myopathy. *Curr Neurol Neurosci Rep*. 2009;9:76–82.

Bushby K. Diagnosis and management of the limb girdle muscular dystrophies. *Pract Neurol*. 2009;9:314–323.

Coiffier L, Perie S, Laforet P, et al. Long-term results of cricopharyngeal myotomy in oculopharyngeal muscular dystrophy. *Otolaryngol Head Neck Surg*. 2006;135:218–222.

Dimachkie MM, Barohn RJ. Guillain-Barré syndrome and variants. *Neurol Clin*. 2013;31:491–510.

Doherty M, Winterton R, Griffiths PG. Eyelid surgery in ocular myopathies. *Orbit*. 2013;32:12–15.

Findlay AR, Goyal NA, Mozaffar T. An overview of polymyositis and dermatomyositis. *Muscle Nerve*. 2015;51:638–656.

Hirano M, Emmanuele V, Quinzii CM. Mitochondrial myopathies. In Tawil RN, Venance S, eds. *Neurology in Practice: Neuromuscular Disorders*. Oxford, UK: Wiley-Blackwell; 2011:42–50. doi:10.1002/9781119973331.ch6

Korner S, Hendricks M, Kollewe K, et al. Weight loss, dysphagia and supplement intake in patients with amyotrophic lateral sclerosis (ALS): impact on quality of life and therapeutic options. *BMC Neurol*. 2013;13:84.

Londral A, Pinto A, Pinto S, et al. Quality of life in amyotrophic lateral sclerosis patients and caregivers: impact of assistive communication from early stages. *Muscle Nerve*. 2015;52:933–941.

Machuca-Tzili L, Brook D, Hilton-Jones D. Clinical and molecular aspects of the myotonic dystrophies: a review. *Muscle Nerve*. 2005;32:1–18.

Manjaly JG, Vaughan-Shaw PG, Dale OT, et al. Cricopharyngeal dilatation for the long-term treatment of dysphagia in oculopharyngeal muscular dystrophy. *Dysphagia*. 2012;27:216–220.

Message banking. https://www.tobiidynavox.com/en-US/software/web-applications/message-banking-2/?MarketPopupClicked=true&utm_medium=referral&utm_source=www.childrenshospital.org

Miller RG, Brooks BR, Swain-Eng RJ, et al. Quality improvement in neurology: amyotrophic lateral sclerosis quality measures: report of the Quality Measurement and Reporting Subcommittee of the American Academy of Neurology. *Neurology*. 2013;81:2136–2140.

Needham M, Mastaglia FL. Sporadic inclusion body myositis: a review of recent clinical advances and current approaches to diagnosis and treatment. *Clin Neurophysiol*. 2016;127:1764–1773.

Phillips PH. Treatment of diplopia. *Semin Neurol*. 2007;27:288–298.

Smith R, Pioro E, Myers K, et al. Enhanced bulbar function in amyotrophic lateral sclerosis: the Nuedexta treatment trial. *Neurotherapeutics*. 2017;14(3):830.

Statland JM, Tawil R. Facioscapulohumeral muscular dystrophy: molecular pathological advances and future directions. *Curr Opin Neurol.* 2011;24:423–428.

Vansteensel MJ, Pels EG, Bleichner MG, et al. Fully implanted brain–computer interface in a locked-in patient with ALS. *N Engl J Med.* 2016;375:2060–2066.

Voice banking. https://www.modeltalker.org

Wang CH, Dowling JJ, North K, et al. Consensus statement on standard of care for congenital myopathies. *J Child Neurol.* 2012;27:363–382.

Wang CH, Finkel RS, Bertini ES, et al. Consensus statement for standard of care in spinal muscular atrophy. *J Child Neurol.* 2007;22:1027–1049.

7 Neuromuscular Respiratory Failure

Nicholas J. Silvestri, Karin Provost, and Daniel W. Sheehan

INTRODUCTION

Respiratory failure is a frequent complication of several neuromuscular disorders that can occur acutely or have a more insidious course. This chapter covers the presenting complaints and physical examination findings in patients with neuromuscular respiratory failure as well as diagnostic studies commonly used in the workup of such patients. It also reviews the differential diagnosis of both acute and chronic neuromuscular respiratory failure and suggested treatment.

PATHOPHYSIOLOGY

To start, a brief review of the pathophysiology of respiratory failure in neuromuscular disorders is warranted (see Figure 7.1). Three main types of physiologic impairment are involved in the development of neuromuscular respiratory failure, which may occur independently, in combination, or in rapid succession with disease progression:

- **Upper airway dysfunction**: Weakness of facial, oropharyngeal, and laryngeal muscles may impair swallowing and clearance of secretions. This increases the risk for aspiration of saliva, liquids, food, and gastroesophageal reflux. It may also result in mechanical obstruction of the upper airway, particularly in the supine position.
- **Inspiratory muscle weakness**: Weakness of the diaphragm, intercostal muscles, and other accessory muscles of respiration leads to impaired ventilation due to impaired lung expansion. The resulting hypoventilation and atelectasis evolves into ventilation/perfusion mismatching, retention of carbon dioxide (CO_2), respiratory acidosis, and eventually hypoxemia. The chronic alveolar hypoventilation often worsens at night with normal sleep-related changes in respiratory physiology; reduced responsiveness to elevations in CO_2 and hypoxia and reduction in tidal volume further exacerbate already impaired ventilatory function.

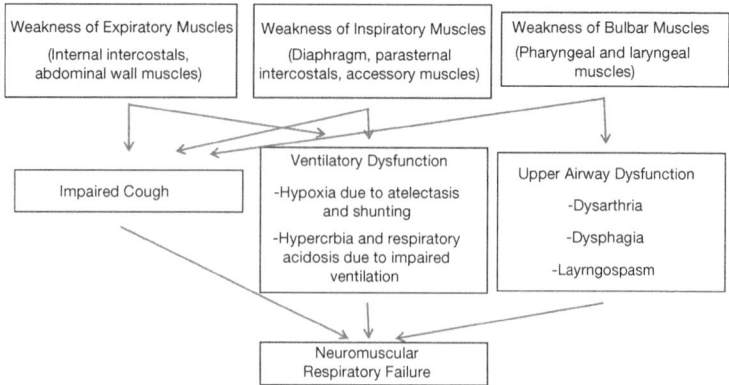

FIGURE 7.1 Pathophysiology of neuromuscular respiratory failure.
Source: Modified from Ref. (1).

- Hypoxia (less than 95% SaO$_2$) is a late manifestation of atelectasis and a sign of impending respiratory failure.
- **Expiratory muscle weakness:** This weakness prevents adequate cough and clearance of airway secretions, also increasing the patient's risk of aspiration.

SYMPTOMS AND SIGNS OF NEUROMUSCULAR RESPIRATORY FAILURE

Symptoms

Patients with chronic alveolar hypoventilation often present with insidious symptoms, before the more overt findings of symptomatic breathlessness (see Table 7.1).

- **EARLY** symptoms relate to progressive hypercapnia, weak coughing, and dysfunctional swallows:
  - Nonrestorative sleep, daytime hypersomnolence
  - Psychological changes or impaired cognitive function (impaired school performance in children)
  - Dyspnea with activities that impair diaphragmatic excursion (bending over, lifting)
  - Orthopnea: limits the ability of gravity to assist diaphragmatic motion (supine or prone positioning, rather than upright)
  - Frequent throat clearing
  - Chest rattle due to retained airway secretions
  - Coughing with eating or drinking
  - Breathy vocal quality due to inability to move sufficient air through the vocal cords

---

TABLE 7.1 Common Symptoms in Neuromuscular Respiratory Failure

Early
Nonrestorative sleep, daytime hypersomnolence
Impaired concentration
Dyspnea with activities that impair diaphragmatic excursion (bending over, lifting)
Orthopnea
Frequent throat clearing
Chest rattle due to retained airway secretions
Coughing with eating or drinking
Breathy vocal quality due to inability to move sufficient air through the vocal cords
Late
Encephalopathy
Dyspnea with exertion
Recurrent pneumonia due to impaired airway clearance and recurrent aspiration

Note: Dyspnea at rest or on exertion with or without concomitant orthopnea is most often due to underlying pulmonary or cardiac disease. A neuromuscular cause for respiratory failure should be suspected once usual pulmonary and cardiac causes of dyspnea have been ruled out or if respiratory symptoms develop in the context of an established neuromuscular illness.

- **LATE** symptoms relate to overt hypercarbic ventilatory failure and respiratory acidosis:
  - Altered mentation and cognition, with marked fatigue due to hypercapnia
  - Dyspnea with exertion due to inability to sustain ventilation sufficiently to meet the physical demands
  - Recurrent pneumonia due to impaired airway clearance and recurrent aspiration

Signs

- Chronic hypoxemia, with oxygen saturation less than 95%
- Elevations in serum bicarbonate levels, reflecting increased renal compensation for chronic hypercapnia and respiratory acidosis
- Rapid, shallow breathing pattern
- Tachycardia
- Use of accessory muscles of respiration
- Difficulty conversing in complete sentences
- Soft, breathy voice
- Anxiety
- Encephalopathy
- Hypoxia upon supine positioning

Defining the Neurologic Etiology of Neuromuscular Respiratory Failure

Once neuromuscular respiratory failure is present, determining the etiology can be challenging.

- Ptosis and/or diplopia, especially if intermittent and worse as the day goes on or with prolonged activity, is suggestive of myasthenia gravis (MG).
- Bifacial weakness can be seen in a number of neuromuscular disorders. If it develops acutely, consideration should be given to Guillain-Barré syndrome (GBS). Patients with certain myopathies, such as type 1 myotonic dystrophy, frequently have facial weakness, referred to as "myopathic facies." Patients with myasthenia may also develop facial weakness.
- Dysphagia can be seen in a range of neuromuscular disorders such as amyotrophic lateral sclerosis (ALS) and MG. Patients with neurogenic dysphagia often first complain of difficulty with consuming liquids more than solids and of frequent coughing during or after meals.
- Dysarthria and dysphonia can also be seen in a number of disorders, including ALS and myasthenia.
- A characteristic feature of myasthenia and other disorders of neuromuscular transmission is fatigability, whereby symptoms tend to worsen the more patients use a particular muscle or group of muscles or as the day goes on.
- Weakness of neck flexors or extensors is an important sign because the degree of weakness in these muscles often parallels weakness of the diaphragm, especially in the acute setting. This sign is frequently seen in ALS, myasthenia, and some myopathies.

The pattern and tempo of limb weakness can help aid in the differential diagnosis:

- Acute (days to weeks)
  - Ascending, symmetrical: GBS, critical illness polyneuropathy (CIP)
  - Descending, symmetrical: botulism, some variants of GBS
  - Proximally predominant, symmetrical: myositis, porphyria, critical illness myopathy (CIM)
  - Oculobulbar-predominant with or without proximal limb involvement: MG, organophosphate poisoning
  - Asymmetrical, affecting named nerves (possibly phrenic): vasculitis, autoimmune brachial plexopathy (e.g., Parsonage-Turner syndrome)
- Subacute to chronic (months to years)
  - Distally predominant at onset, asymmetrical: ALS, multifocal motor neuropathy (MMN)

- ▪ Proximally predominant at onset, often symmetrical: muscular dystrophies, inflammatory and metabolic myopathies (e.g., Pompe disease)

In addition to weakness, other symptoms and signs are helpful:

- Muscle atrophy is common in ALS.
- Fasciculations are common in motor neuron disorders (e.g., tongue fasciculations in SMA type 1, ALS).
- Sensory symptoms may include numbness, paresthesias, and neuropathic pain in GBS and in central causes (e.g., cord compression or myelitis).
- Bowel/bladder dysfunction may be seen in GBS as well as spinal cord pathology.
- Signs of dysautonomia are frequently seen in GBS and botulism.
- Hyperreflexia is commonly seen in ALS but also may be seen with cord pathology. Areflexia is a common early sign in GBS.

A history of possible precipitants for respiratory failure is important to ascertain:

- Recent infections, especially upper respiratory tract infections and diarrheal illnesses, are reported in two-thirds of cases of GBS 2 to 3 weeks before the development of neurologic symptoms. In addition, upper respiratory tract infections may precipitate acute respiratory failure in patients with chronic neuromuscular disorders such as ALS, MG, and Duchenne muscular dystrophy (DMD).
- Recent vaccinations or trauma have been reported to precipitate GBS.
- A history of starting a new medication or a dose increase in a medication may be important. Certain medications may lead to weakness (e.g., 3-hydroxy-3-methyl-glutaryl-coenzyme A [HMG-CoA] reductase inhibitors or "statins") and many can cause an exacerbation in patients with MG.
- Toxin exposures—for example, organophosphates, heavy metal toxicity.
- Systemic symptoms: Are there clues from the history that might suggest the presence of an underlying medical illness that might have neurologic sequelae (e.g., vasculitis)?
- Prior history: Is there a prior history of symptoms that might point to a diagnosis? For example, patients with MG often have a transient history of mild ptosis and or diplopia months before they develop more severe symptoms.
- Family history: Is there a known family history of a neurologic disorder? For example, DMD is X-linked, 10% of cases of ALS are familial, and autoimmune disorders tend to cluster in families.

CLINICAL INVESTIGATION

Laboratory: General Screening

- Complete blood count (CBC) and comprehensive metabolic profile (CMP) are important to evaluate for an underlying metabolic derangement that may have precipitated respiratory failure.
- Electrolyte abnormalities: Hyperkalemia or hypokalemia, hypercalcemia or hypocalcemia, hypermagnesemia, and hypophosphatemia may all cause acute generalized weakness with respiratory failure.
- Creatine kinase (CK) is often very elevated in myopathies—early in muscular dystrophies and acutely in inflammatory myopathies. Less severe increases in CK may be seen in ALS.
- Arterial, venous, or capillary blood gas evaluation is necessary to determine the presence and severity of CO_2 retention and respiratory acidosis. Pulse oximetry is insensitive to detect hypoventilation and respiratory acidosis. In pure hypoventilation, arterial PCO_2 can be 50 mmHg or higher when oxygen-hemoglobin saturations (SpO_2) are in the range of 94% to 95%. Supplemental oxygen can maintain SpO_2 in the 95% to 100% range, with PCO_2 above 60 mmHg.
- Infectious evaluation.

Laboratory Testing: Specific Neurologic Causes

- Acetylcholine receptor antibodies (AChR Abs) are found in 85% of patients with generalized MG. These antibodies are usually of the binding type, but rare patients may have blocking or modulating antibodies. Roughly 7% of patients with generalized myasthenia have antibodies to muscle receptor tyrosine kinase (MuSK). Patients with MuSK antibodies more often have bulbar-predominant weakness and are prone to episodes of respiratory failure known as myasthenic crises.
- Acid maltase deficiency should be suspected in patients with otherwise unexplained neuromuscular respiratory failure with or without proximal muscle weakness. Testing for acid maltase deficiency can be done utilizing a dried blood spot test and confirmed with appropriate genetic testing.
- Analysis of cerebrospinal fluid (CSF): The classic albuminocytologic dissociation (normal white blood cell [WBC] count with elevation in protein) is seen in over 80% of patients with GBS within 2 weeks of symptom onset. It is important to note that CSF protein may be normal in up to one-third of patients in the first week of this disease. Elevation of WBCs in the CSF should raise concern for an infectious or inflammatory etiology, and the clinical context must be taken into account. For example, with an elevation in WBC count in a patient with rapidly ascending weakness

mimicking GBS, consideration should be given to HIV, Lyme disease, and sarcoidosis. If the patient presents with encephalopathy and asymmetric limb weakness and wasting, a disorder such as West Nile virus poliomyelitis is on the differential diagnosis.

Advanced Diagnostic Studies

- **Magnetic resonance imaging (MRI)** of the brain or cervical spine should be considered in any patient with long tract signs.
- **Electrodiagnostic testing** is helpful in identifying specific neurologic causes of respiratory failure.

A detailed review of nerve conduction studies and electromyography can be found in Chapter 1. Table 7.2 highlights findings that may be seen in disorders frequently leading to neuromuscular respiratory failure.

- **Muscle biopsy:** In general, muscle biopsy is of limited utility in the case of acute neuromuscular respiratory failure. It might be helpful if inflammatory myopathy is suspected, or in the case of critical illness myopathy where one will see loss of thick (myosin) filaments. Combined muscle and nerve biopsy are also useful in the case of suspected vasculitis with phrenic nerve involvement.

Pulmonary Function Testing (PFT)—Diagnostic

- A restrictive pattern may be seen on full PFT. Spirometry alone is insufficient, but can be suggestive if the FEV_1 (forced expiratory volume in 1 second) and the forced vital capacity (FVC) are equally or nearly equally reduced and less than 80% predicted. Low MIP and MEP differentiate neuromuscular respiratory failure from other causes of restrictive lung diseases.
- A drop in FVC or vital capacity (VC) of more than 10% from upright to supine positioning indicates diaphragmatic dysfunction.*
- Negative inspiratory force/maximum inspiratory pressure (NIF/MIP) is a good indicator of diaphragmatic function. Normal is less than or equal to 70 cm H_2O. For full inspiration, at least –40 cm H_2O is needed.
- Maximum expiratory pressure (MEP) is a good indicator of expiratory force/cough function. Normal is more than 100 cm H_2O. Cough is likely ineffective when MEP less than 60 cm H_2O.
- Peak cough flow of less than 270 L/min is suggestive of ineffective cough.*
- Reduced VC of less than 25 mL/kg.*

The single breath count test involves asking a patient to count out loud on one continuous expiration after a long inspiration. In a normal single breath count test, the patient can count to at least 50 on

---

*Tests can be done at the bedside, for rapid assessment of respiratory status.

TABLE 7.2 Electrodiagnostic Findings in Common Causes of Neuromuscular Respiratory Failure

Condition	CMAP	SNAP	EMG spontaneous activity	EMG motor unit morphology	EMG recruitment	Slow (3 Hz) RNS	Fast (50 Hz) RNS
Amyotrophic lateral sclerosis	NI or ↓amplitude NI CV	NI	++	↑amplitude ↑duration polyphasic	→	NI	NI
Guillain-Barré syndrome	NI or ↓amplitude Slowed CV and prolonged distal latencies	NI or ↓amplitude Slowed CV and prolonged latencies	NI	NI	→	NI	NI
Critical illness polyneuropathy	↓amplitudes NI CV	↓amplitudes NI CV	+	↑amplitude ↑duration polyphasic	→	NI	NI
Myasthenia gravis	NI	NI	NI	NI	NI	Abnormal	NI
Lambert-Eaton myasthenic syndrome	↓amplitude NI CV	NI	NI	NI	NI	NI	Abnormal
Botulism	↓amplitude NI CV	NI	NI	++	NI	NI	Abnormal

(continued)

TABLE 7.2 Electrodiagnostic Findings in Common Causes of Neuromuscular Respiratory Failure (*continued*)

Condition	CMAP	SNAP	EMG spontaneous activity	EMG motor unit morphology	EMG recruitment	Slow (3 Hz) RNS	Fast (50 Hz) RNS
Critical illness myopathy	↓amplitude NI CV	NI	+	↓amplitude ↓duration polyphasic	Early	NI	NI
Acid maltase deficiency	NI	NI	++ Myotonia	NI or ↓amplitude ↓duration polyphasic	NI	NI	NI
Inflammatory myopathies	↓amplitude NI CV	NI	++	↓amplitude ↓duration polyphasic	Early	NI	NI

CMAP, compound motor action potential; CV, conduction velocity; EMG, electromyography; NI, normal; SNAP, sensory nerve action potential.

one breath; counting to less than 15 is concerning for impairment in FVC. The number a person is able to count to roughly parallels FVC.*

Pulmonary Function Testing: Determination of Need for Respiratory Support Devices

The "20-30-40-50-60" rule:

- MEP <**60** cm H_2O (or PCF<270 L/min): airway clearance (mechanical insufflator/exsufflator)
- FVC <**50**%: nocturnal noninvasive ventilatory support
- MEP <**40** cm H_2O: daytime noninvasive ventilatory support
- MIP <**30** cm H_2O: daytime noninvasive ventilatory support
- VC <**20** mL/kg: likely dependent on ventilatory support
- In their study on predictors of respiratory failure in GBS, Lawn et al. found that progression to mechanical ventilation was more likely to occur in patients with rapid disease progression, bulbar involvement, bifacial weakness, or dysautonomia. They also found that factors associated with the development of respiratory failure on PFTs included FVC <20 cc/kg, MIP <30 cm H_2O, MEP <40 cm H_2O, or a reduction of more than 30% of baseline measurements at the time of presentation in these parameters.
- The frequency of serial monitoring of FVCs depends on the nature of the respiratory failure: acute versus chronic.
- Walgaard et al. developed a predictive model to assess at the time of admission the likelihood of development of respiratory failure at 1 week in patients with GBS. This model is termed the Erasmus GBS Respiratory Insufficiency Score (EGRIS) and takes into account the rate of disease progression, the Medical Research Council (MRC) sum score, and the presence of facial or bulbar weakness. The eight-point score adequately predicts the eventual need for mechanical ventilation, ranging from 1% to 90%.

DIFFERENTIAL DIAGNOSIS

Figure 7.2 provides an algorithm for the differential diagnosis of acute generalized weakness and neuromuscular respiratory failure.

Central Causes

- Lesions of the medulla may affect the nuclei critical for normal breathing, including demyelinating, neoplastic, infectious, and vascular processes. Ondine's curse (central hypoventilation syndrome) is a rare disorder that may be either congenital or acquired and affects automatic breathing, sparing voluntary breathing. It often manifests as respiratory failure during sleep.

---

*Tests can be done at the bedside, for rapid assessment of respiratory status.

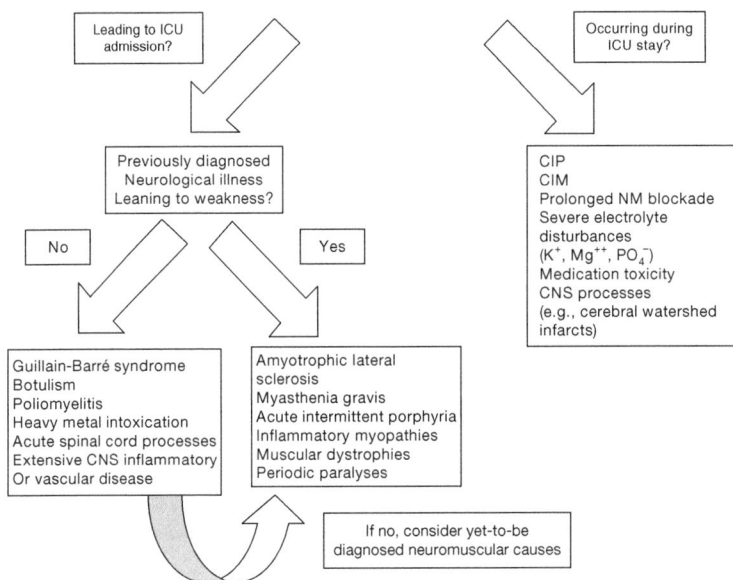

FIGURE 7.2 Diagnostic algorithm for determining cause of generalized weakness and/or failure to wean from the ventilator.

CIM, critical illness myopathy; CIP, critical illness polyneuropathy, CNS, central nervous system.

- Lesions of the high cervical cord at or above the C3 to C5 level may cause respiratory failure, as the diaphragm is innervated by these nerve roots. Trauma, myelitis (e.g., due to multiple sclerosis or neuromyeliltis optica), and neoplasms are all considerations.

Anterior Horn

- ALS: Respiratory dysfunction occurs in almost all cases of ALS at some point in the disease and can be an early symptom leading to diagnosis. The most common causes of death in ALS are respiratory failure and pneumonia.
- Spinal muscular atrophy (SMA): Respiratory dysfunction occurs early in SMA type 1 (the first few months of life), later in SMA type 2, and rarely in SMA types 3 and 4.
- West Nile virus (WNV)–related poliomyelitis: WNV most often causes a self-limited flu-like illness but severe cases can progress to meningitis, encephalitis, and even more rarely poliomyelitis. The weakness in these cases is often asymmetrical with a predilection for proximal muscles, and diaphragmatic involvement has been described.
- Kennedy's disease (X-linked bulbospinal muscular atrophy): Progressive respiratory failure may occur in this disorder as in ALS.

Nerve

- GBS: GBS is the most common cause of acute flaccid paralysis, with an estimated annual incidence of 2 per 100,000. It causes the rapid progression of weakness and sensory symptoms, usually in an ascending pattern over the course of days to weeks. Respiratory failure occurs in approximately 30% of patients with GBS and is associated with a poor functional outcome. The median duration of mechanical ventilation is 20 to 30 days and the mortality in mechanically ventilated patients as high as 20%. Quadriplegia, older age, the presence of multiple medical comorbidities, and more severe axonal changes on electrodiagnostic studies are predictive of longer duration of mechanical ventilation. Dysautonomia occurs in roughly two-thirds of patients with GBS and may lead to the need for mechanical ventilation if hemodynamic instability is severe. Treatment with intravenous immunoglobulin (IVIG) or plasma exchange may reduce the duration of mechanical ventilation.

- MMN: Respiratory failure in this disorder is rare but can occur with phrenic nerve involvement.

- Charcot-Marie-Tooth (CMT) disease: Chronic respiratory failure has been reported in several CMT variants but in general respiratory failure is rare.

- CIP: This disorder is especially common in patients in the ICU with sepsis; it occurs in 50% to 70% of patients with systemic inflammatory response syndrome (SIRS), according to several studies. CIP is often accompanied by septic encephalopathy, making adequate assessment of strength and sensation difficult. It is a generalized severe sensorimotor polyneuropathy that spares the cranial nerves but has frequent phrenic nerve involvement. The diagnosis is typically made when patients who survive sepsis have difficulty weaning from mechanical ventilation. The average duration of mechanical ventilation in patients with CIP in one study was 34 days, versus 14 days for those without CIP, in a cohort of critically ill patients.

- Other rare forms of neuropathy that may lead to respiratory failure include heavy metal toxicity (arsenic, thallium, lead), porphyria, and vasculitis with phrenic nerve involvement.

- Phrenic nerve injury can occur as a result of trauma, direct compression from adjacent structures, or infiltration by malignancy or metastases, or it may be inflammatory in nature (including involvement in Parsonage-Turner syndrome). If the injury is unilateral, patients may complain of platypnea (difficulty breathing when lying on their side); if it is bilateral, they may complain of orthopnea and dyspnea at rest. The radiographic sniff test or ultrasound can be helpful in determining the presence of diaphragmatic weakness.

Neuromuscular Junction

- MG: Respiratory failure in MG is termed myasthenic crisis and occurs in 15% to 20% of patients with this disease at some point in their illness. Myasthenic crisis can be the presenting symptom of the disease in 15% of patients, or it can occur in patients with a known diagnosis and acute worsening. The risk for crisis is highest in the first 3 years after diagnosis and is usually associated with worsening of ocular, bulbar, neck, and limb strength. In about 70% of cases, crisis is precipitated by an illness, infection, new medication (e.g., aminoglycosides or high-dose corticosteroids), stress, or another provocative factor. The median duration of mechanical ventilation in myasthenic crisis is 14 days, with age older than 50, pre-intubation serum bicarbonate level greater than 30 mEq/L, and peak vital capacity less than 25 cc/kg at 1 to 6 days post-intubation being risk factors for the need for mechanical ventilation lasting more than 2 weeks. Treatment is directed against any identified precipitants, such as infection, and against the disease with plasma exchange. Mortality in myasthenic crisis is less than 5% and is usually due to complications.

- Lambert-Eaton myasthenic syndrome (LEMS): Respiratory failure is rare in LEMS but has been reported in the literature.

- Botulism: Poisoning with botulinum toxin can cause the rapid progression of weakness, autonomic instability, and respiratory failure that may mimic either GBS or MG. Respiratory failure can often be predicted by the presence of signs of autonomic dysfunction, including urinary retention and emesis. The duration of mechanical ventilation is often several months while slow recovery occurs.

- Prolonged neuromuscular blockade: This disorder is rare and is usually seen in patients with liver or renal failure who are treated with neuromuscular blocking agents so as to facilitate mechanical ventilation. It may mimic MG and is self-limited once the offending agents have been metabolized.

- Other neuromuscular disorders leading to respiratory failure include certain forms of tick paralysis, poisoning with various forms of venom, organophosphate poisoning, and hypermagnesemia.

Muscle

- CIM: This relatively rapidly progressive myopathy is seen in patients treated in the ICU and is linked with use of high-dose corticosteroids and neuromuscular blocking agents. As there is frequent involvement of the cranial nerves and diaphragm, respiratory failure is a common symptom. Like CIP, CIM is associated with a longer duration of mechanical ventilation and difficulty weaning from the ventilator. The recovery tends to be quicker in CIM than in CIP.

- DMD: Respiratory failure begins as early as the teen years, with gradual decline usually leading to death in the second to third decade.
- Respiratory failure has also been described in the following muscular dystrophies: sarcoglycanopathies (limb-girdle muscular dystrophy types 2C, 2D, 2E, and 2F), congenital muscular dystrophy type 1A (merosin deficiency), facioscapulohumeral muscular dystrophy (less than 1% of patients), and Bethlem myopathy.
- Acid maltase deficiency (Pompe disease): Respiratory failure is the leading cause of death in infantile Pompe disease and in the juvenile form, in which progressive weakness of the ventilatory muscles typically leads to death in the second or third decade. In the adult-onset form, there is also frequent involvement of muscles of respiration, such that up to one-third of patients first present with respiratory dysfunction before the development of the more characteristic proximal muscle weakness. This is an important disorder to diagnose, as it is treatable with enzyme replacement therapy.
- Inflammatory myopathies: Respiratory dysfunction can occur in severe cases of polymyositis and dermatomyositis, usually in the context of severe generalized weakness.
- Congenital myopathies: Multi/minicore myopathy, nemaline myopathy, X-linked centronuclear/myotubular myopathy, congenital fiber-type disproportion, and reducing body myopathy are all congenital myopathies associated with varying degrees of respiratory dysfunction.

MANAGEMENT OF NEUROMUSCULAR RESPIRATORY FAILURE

This section focuses on the management of neuromuscular respiratory failure from a pulmonary perspective. Disease-specific management (e.g., the treatment of GBS and MG) are covered elsewhere in this book.

Acute Respiratory Failure

Supplemental oxygen should **not** be used without first supporting ventilation. Supplemental oxygen can suppress ventilation in individuals who chronically retain CO_2. Respiratory acidosis can be reversed with noninvasive ventilation delivered via bilevel positive airway pressure (BiPAP) or volume ventilator (assured volume averaged pressure support [AVAPS], continuous mandatory ventilation [CMV] with sip ventilation). Possible interfaces include nasal pillows, nasal mask, mouthpiece, and full face mask. Full face mask ventilation should not be used if patients are at high risk of aspiration, vomiting, or gastroesophageal reflux. Noninvasive ventilation with a backup rate of 16 to 24 breaths per minute will most often prevent the need for intubation, both acutely as an inpatient and with chronic outpatient respiratory insufficiency.

- Typical bilevel pressures are inspiratory pressures (IPAP) of 14 to 22 cm H_2O; expiratory pressures (EPAP) of 4 to 6 cm H_2O are most comfortable for individuals with weak expiratory muscles.
- For noninvasive volume ventilation (NIV), tidal volumes (VT) of 7 to 10 cc/kg or 500 to 700 mL are typically needed.
- Mechanical cough assistance with a mechanical insufflator/exsufflator (MI/E; "cough assist") can also clear lower airway secretions and reverse hypoxemia, hypercapnia, and respiratory acidosis. To simulate a cough, typical MI/E pressures are +40 cm H_2O for inspiration and –40 cm H_2O on expiration. MI/E is used at least every 4 hours, when a chest/throat rattle is heard or palpated, and whenever there is an acute drop in SpO_2 to less than 95%. The most effective airway clearance treatment options are MI/E and intermittent positive-pressure breathing with manually assisted cough.

If noninvasive ventilation is not effective in reversing acute respiratory acidosis, then intubation is warranted for adequate ventilation. Using minimal or no supplemental oxygen is helpful in determining whether as needed (prn) MI/E is needed in pneumonia—that is, if SpO_2 falls to less than 95%, MI/E is warranted to clear the airway secretions causing desaturations.

Nutrition should be optimized, and fasting/NPO (nothing by mouth) restrictions should be avoided to prevent catabolism and further muscle weakening.

Attempts to wean or sprint intubated patients with neuromuscular disorders can lead to fatigue, further weakness, and atelectasis and is not recommended. Per the extubation protocol described by Bach et al. (2), extubation to full support noninvasive ventilation should be considered when SpO_2 is 95% or greater on room air, chest x-ray is clear or near clear, and the patient is fully alert and cooperative and not receiving sedatives. This extubation protocol has a first attempt extubation success rate of 95% even in "unweanable" patients. Full support noninvasive ventilation settings for successful extubations are as follows: assist control, volume of 800 to 1500 mL in adults, pressure control of at least 18 cm H_2O and rate of 10 to 14 breaths per minute.

If three attempts of this protocol fail, tracheostomy should be discussed with the patient, healthcare proxy, and care providers. Palliative care consults should be considered early in intensive care admissions.

Chronic Respiratory Failure

Patients with chronic respiratory failure can be supported with noninvasive ventilatory support 24 hours a day (e.g., nasal or full face mask ventilation when asleep; nasal or mouthpiece sip volume ventilation when awake). Full face mask ventilation should not be used if patients are at high risk of aspiration, vomiting, or gastro-esophageal reflux. Noninvasive ventilation will improve quality of life and treat the respiratory insufficiency, leading to prolonged survival and slowing of the rate of FVC decline. Although NIV does not increase survival in bulbar predominant disorders (ALS), it does improve quality of life and should still be offered.

Invasive ventilation (tracheostomy/ventilator) should be considered when bulbar weakness leads to salivary aspiration; noninvasive ventilation is inadequate despite optimization; or patients and caregivers prefer this technique. Prior to considering tracheostomy placement, consultation with palliative care or advanced illness support teams should be strongly considered, to explore the

---

BEFORE EXTUBATION:
For **INTUBATED** patients, q 4 hours airway clearance AND prn Cough Assist:
1. Cough assist: 5 sets of 5 breaths;

Inspiratory pressure:	+35 or +40	for	2 seconds;
Expiratory pressure:	-35 or -40	for	2 seconds;
Pause:	2 seconds		

2. ETT suctioning followed by BAGGING.
3. Vest therapy or chest PT for 20 to 30 minutes.
4. Cough assist: 5 sets of 5 breaths as above; **end on inspiration to re-expand**
5. ETT suctioning followed by BAGGING

> **Use Cough Assist if O_2 sat drops to < 95% acutely**

* Cough assist can be used every 10 minutes followed by ETT suctioning and BAGGING.

CONSIDER EXTUBATION when the patient is:
- Afebrile
- **NOT** requiring supplemental O_2.
- CXR is without atelectasis or infiltrates
- Off all respiratory depressants
- Minimal secretions.

"SPRINTING" OR CPAP TRIALS ARE NOT RECOMMENDED
- They can result in atelectasis and fatigue.
- While the patient is intubated, wean to home or full nasal ventilation settings.

AFTER EXTUBATION:
EXTUBATE to home or full nasal ventilation settings and **NO** supplemental O_2.
(e.g., BiPap of (14–20)/(3–6) using spontaneous timed mode; backup rate = spontaneous rate)

After **EXTUBATION**, minimum of q 4 hours airway clearance AND prn Cough Assist as above.
Expect frequent Cough Assist for first 1-2 hours after EXTUBATION.

> **Use Cough Assist if O_2 sats drops to <95% acutely**

Wean from nasal BiPap or ventilation during the day as tolerated.

FIGURE 7.3 Recommended protocol for extubation of patients with chronic neuromuscular respiratory failure.

Source: Modified from Refs. (2,3).

patient and caregiver understanding of disease, and define goals of care. Recommendations for the postoperative care of patients with chronic neuromuscular disorders are shown in Figure 7.3.

REFERENCES

1. Benditt JO, Boitano LJ. Pulmonary issues in patients with chronic neuromuscular disease. *Am J Respir Crit Care Med*. 2013;187(10):1046–1055.
2. Bach JR, Goncalves MR, Hamdani I, Winck JC. Extubation of patients with neuromuscular weakness: a new management paradigm. *Chest*. 2010;137(5):1033–1039.
3. Bach JR, Niranjan V, Weaver B. Spinal muscular atrophy type 1: a noninvasive respiratory management approach. *Chest*. 2000;117(4):1100–1105.

SUGGESTED READING

Bach JR, Gonçalves MR, Hon A, et al. Changing trends in the management of end-stage neuromuscular respiratory muscle failure: recommendations of an international consensus. *Am J Phys Med Rehabil*. 2013;92(3):267–277.

Bolton CF. Neuromuscular manifestations of critical illness. *Muscle Nerve*. 2005;32:140–163.

Bourke SC, Tomlinson M, Williams TL, et al. Effects of non-invasive ventilation on survival and quality of life in patients with amyotrophic lateral sclerosis: a randomised controlled trial. *Lancet Neurol*. 2006;5(2):140–147.

Brasil Santos D, Vaugier I, Boussaïd G, et al. Impact of noninvasive ventilation on lung volumes and maximum respiratory pressures in Duchenne muscular dystrophy. *Respir Care*. 2016;61(11):1530–1535.

Carratù P, Spicuzza L, Cassano A, et al. Early treatment with noninvasive positive pressure ventilation prolongs survival in amyotrophic lateral sclerosis patients with nocturnal respiratory insufficiency. *Orphanet J Rare Dis*. 2009;4:10.

Fu E, Downs JB, Schweiger JW, et al. Supplemental oxygen impairs detection of hypoventilation by pulse oximetry. *Chest*. 2004;126(5):1552–1558.

Gruis K, Lechtzin N. Respiratory therapies for amyotrophic lateral sclerosis: a primer muscle nerve. *Muscle Nerve*. 2012;46(3): 313–331.

Hardiman O. Management of respiratory symptoms in ALS. *J Neurol*. 2011;258:359–365.

Homnick DN. Mechanical insufflation-exsufflation for airway mucus clearance. *Respir Care*. 2007;52(10):1296–1305.

Lawn ND, Fletcher DD, Henderson RD, et al. Anticipating mechanical ventilation in Guillain-Barré syndrome. *Arch Neurol.* 2001;58(6):893–898.

McKim DA, Griller N, LeBlanc C, et al. Twenty-four hour noninvasive ventilation in Duchenne muscular dystrophy: a safe alternative to tracheostomy. *Can Respir J.* 2013;20(1):e5–e9.

Walgaard C, Lingsma HF, Ruts L, et al. Prediction of respiratory insufficiency in Guillain-Barré syndrome. *Ann Neurol.* 2010;67:781–787.

8 Sensory Loss and Neuropathic Pain

Kelly G. Gwathmey and Nora Jovanovich

This chapter covers various conditions that primarily affect the sensory components of the nervous system, including small and large nerve fibers, dorsal root ganglia (DRG), and the trigeminal nerve. Understanding of normal structure and function of the sensory nervous system serves as a framework for understanding dysfunction caused by damage to the various components.

To review, two primary sensory pathways transmit information to the brain.

- The first transmits thermal and nociceptive inputs, while the second transmits light touch, vibratory, and proprioceptive inputs.
  - In this pathway, small myelinated Aδ fibers and unmyelinated C fibers arrive at the large light and small dark cell bodies respectively, both of which are housed in the DRG. These small neurons relay information about pain and temperature to the brain via the spinothalamic tracts. Additionally, Aδ fibers help to regulate preganglionic sympathetic and parasympathetic systems while C fibers help to regulate the postganglionic autonomic system.
- In the second pathway, Aβ fibers arrive at the large light cell bodies within the DRG and continue via posterior columns of the spinal cord to transmit vibratory, proprioceptive, and tactile information to the brain.
- The trigeminal nerve is the largest of the cranial nerves and carries sensory input not only from the face but also from the dura mater, nasal, oral, and sinus mucosa. The three main branches of the trigeminal nerve are the ophthalmic (V1), maxillary (V2), and mandibular (V3). The mandibular division also carries efferent motor fibers to the muscles of mastication.
- Impaired function of the small myelinated and unmyelinated, large fibers, DRG, and trigeminal nerves causes distinct clinical presentations that are discussed in detail in this chapter. Emphasis is placed on formulating a differential diagnosis based on

localization determined by clinical symptoms and focused physical examination. The necessary laboratory testing, electrodiagnostic testing, and tissue biopsy to support various diagnoses are also discussed. Finally, symptomatic management and disease-specific treatments are reviewed.

HISTORY

Patients can present with a range of symptoms referable to the sensory component of the nervous system.

- It is best to consider first if a patient has a neuropathic pain-predominant presentation supporting small fiber localization versus an ataxia-predominant presentation suggesting localization to the large nerve fibers, DRG, and dorsal columns.
- Patients may also present with painless sensory loss with preserved ambulation, supporting either localization to the large fibers in the distal extremities or a painless form of small fiber neuropathy.
- In patients with focal sensory complaints such as a single dermatome or a portion of the face, the localization may be a single dorsal root ganglion or a division of the trigeminal nerve, respectively. These patients will present quite differently from those who have a more widespread sensory polyneuropathy.
- When encountering a patient with sensory complaints, it is of paramount importance to determine the tempo of the presentation. The differential diagnoses for acute and chronic sensory neuropathic symptoms are quite separate.
- An appreciation of the pattern of symptoms (e.g., localized, length-dependent, generalized, multifocal) will guide the physician to an appropriate differential diagnosis. The fundamental features of different sensory presentations follow.

Small Fiber Presentation

Patients presenting with small fiber-mediated dysfunction complain of positive or negative neuropathic symptoms.

- Positive neuropathic symptoms are described as "electrical," "shooting," "burning," and "tingling." Spontaneous stimulus-independent pain due to nociceptor C-fiber activity occurs.
- Stimulus-evoked pain is interpreted as either allodynia or hyperalgesia.
  - Allodynia occurs when a non-noxious stimulus is interpreted as painful. Hyperalgesia occurs when a patient perceives a painful stimulus as even more painful. This is hypothesized to be the result of abnormal processing of nociceptor input. Neuropathic pain often worsens at night and prevents or disrupts sleep. Patients complain of the bedsheets or their socks causing discomfort. High temperatures will also trigger pain.

- Negative neuropathic symptoms are reported as a "loss of sensation" or "numbness." Patients express a "bunched-up sock feeling" on the soles of their feet. The patients do not typically complain of weakness or gait imbalance, but may state that walking is painful.
- Patients with small fiber neuropathies usually describe a length-dependent or "stocking/glove" pattern. Symptoms start in their toes and spread rostrally.
- When patients complain of generalized or non-length-dependent numbness and neuropathic pain affecting their face, arms, and trunk, autoimmune and metabolic diseases should be highly considered.
- Many patients with small fiber dysfunction will have involvement of their autonomic nervous system. We highly recommend basic autonomic screening questions for any patient referred for a question of neuropathy.
  - Eliciting a history of significant autonomic impairment helps with narrowing the differential diagnosis and may direct further workup.
  - Symptoms of autonomic dysfunction include hypohidrosis (often in the distal extremities), hyperhidrosis (often in the trunk and proximal extremities), dry eyes, dry mouth, orthostatic dizziness, palpitations, gastroparesis, urinary retention, erectile dysfunction, constipation, and skin discoloration.

Large Fiber and Sensory Ataxia Presentations

Patients with classic large fiber neuropathies develop a length-dependent loss of sensation, which over time may result in sensory ataxia due to impaired proprioception.

- Disorders of the large sensory fibers do not typically occur in isolation. Thus, patients will also complain of positive sensory symptoms resulting from dysfunction of the $A\delta$ and C fibers.
- Patients with severe, large fiber dysfunction localizing to the DRG (sensory neuronopathies or dorsal root ganglionopathies) or the dorsal columns of the spinal cord will have early gait imbalance and incoordination. Patients will complain of frequent tripping and falls and may present in a wheelchair. These patients report multifocal, non-length-dependent positive or negative sensory symptoms in a patchy distribution over the arms, legs, and trunk. Patients may also have facial involvement if the trigeminal ganglia are affected.
- Depending on the cause of the large fiber sensory nerve impairment, patients may report weakness due to involvement of the motor nerves or anterior horn cells. Many patients with length-dependent large fiber sensory neuropathies will develop

distal extremity weakness over time. Weakness is not a feature of the purest sensory neuronopathies, as destruction is isolated to the DRG, but damage to the motor nerves and anterior horn cells may occur depending on the etiology (i.e., paraneoplastic).

Localized Sensory Symptoms

- Patients presenting with localized sensory complaints fall into an entirely separate category. Some of the most frequently encountered patients are those presenting with symptoms localizing to an individual peripheral nerve. For example, the patient who presents to the clinic with hand numbness and tingling in the first, second, and third digits likely has carpal tunnel syndrome caused by a median mononeuropathy at the wrist. A full review of the various mononeuropathies that present with sensory complaints is beyond the scope of this chapter and is reviewed elsewhere, as these conditions often have accompanying motor deficits. Other causes of focal sensory symptoms will localize to an individual dermatome (nerve root and associated dorsal root ganglion) and the trigeminal nerve. These presentations are covered briefly in this chapter.

- When patients present with neuropathic pain and sensory disturbance in an isolated dermatome, they often have associated neck or low back pain, suggesting an underlying cervical or lumbosacral radiculopathy affecting primarily the sensory fibers of the nerve root. These patients complain of radiating or shooting pain that travels down their arm or leg. This pain worsens with the Valsalva maneuver (e.g., cough, sneeze) due to the transient increase in intraspinal pressure. The other common condition is shingles (acute herpes zoster infection) and the resultant postherpetic neuralgia, which usually affects a single thoracic or lumbar dermatome or the ophthalmic division of the trigeminal nerve (zoster ophthalmicus or zoster keratitis). Patients complain of a deep burning, stabbing pain that may be constant or occur spontaneously. Superimposed on this pain is stimulus-evoked pain (allodynia and hyperalgesia).

- Another cause of neuropathic facial pain is trigeminal neuralgia. Patients with trigeminal neuralgia complain of stereotyped paroxysms of sharp, stabbing pain in the distribution of the trigeminal nerve (typically V2 or V3 distributions). The electrical pain may last only seconds, but recurs over and over. Eventually there may become a dull pain between the paroxysms. Reported triggers of trigeminal neuralgia include cold air, brushing teeth, and chewing. On rare occasions, patients may present with facial numbness that is localized to the trigeminal nerve or one of its divisions. When the numbness predominates, a diagnosis of trigeminal neuropathy should be considered.

Context

When interviewing a patient with sensory complaints, it imperative to understand the context in which the symptoms developed.

- Vitamin deficiencies occur due to insufficient intake or malabsorption, and malnutrition will be evident from the patient's history. Those with eating disorders or strict adherence to a vegan diet are most at risk. Malabsorption occurs due to a variety of factors. Vitamin B_{12} malabsorption can occur due to impaired binding of intrinsic factor to vitamin B_{12} for various reasons, including atrophic gastritis due to prolonged antacid use (proton-pump inhibitor or H_2-antagonists), gastric bypass, or damage or resection of the terminal ileum in the setting of Crohn's disease. Copper also is absorbed in the stomach and small bowel, so its malabsorption may arise due to gastric or intestinal surgery. Because zinc toxicity prevents absorption of copper, zinc levels should be checked as part of the malabsorption workup. A complete blood count (CBC) to evaluate for anemia is helpful as well. Vitamin E deficiency usually occurs only with severe fat malabsorption as seen with profound biliary dysfunction, cystic fibrosis, or abetalipoproteinemia, a genetic disorder. Vitamin B_6 is abundantly available from dietary sources and its malabsorption is rare. Deficiencies usually result from isoniazid treatment for tuberculosis or, rarely, gastric bypass surgery.
- Asking a patient if he or she has diabetes is of clear value given the association between diabetes and neuropathy. If the patient denies carrying that diagnosis, inquiring about polydipsia, polyuria, and weight loss may alert the physician that the patient has undiagnosed diabetes or may have impaired glucose tolerance.
- Asking the patient about systemic symptoms such as night sweats, weight loss, rash, joint pain, or other organ involvement may guide the physician to a neoplastic or autoimmune etiology. In contrast, a history of exposure to a neurotoxic drug (frequently chemotherapeutic agents) suggests a toxic neuropathy.
- A strong family history of similar sensory complaints and foot deformities suggests an inherited etiology. If affected family members are present at the appointment, examination of their feet may reveal the diagnosis.

CLINICAL INVESTIGATIONS

Examination Findings

After taking a detailed history, a comprehensive physical exam helps guide the clinical investigation.

- The examination of patients with a small fiber-predominant presentation will often reveal dry, discolored, and shiny atrophic skin of their distal lower extremities due to impaired distal autonomic vasomotor control.

- Pain (tested with pinprick) and temperature sensation is impaired in a length-dependent or non-length-dependent fashion. In patients with a pure small fiber neuropathy, large fiber-mediated sensation (vibratory sensation and proprioception), strength, and deep tendon reflexes will be spared. As a result, patients will not have gait ataxia, though their gait may appear antalgic.
- If the history is suggestive of a large fiber sensory-predominant neuropathy, neurologic examination can help to support this diagnosis. Vibration, proprioception, or light touch sensation may be diminished or absent. If small fiber sensation is also affected, pinprick sensation may be heightened, diminished, or absent. Involvement of the large fiber sensory nerves in the extremities usually leads to altered sensation in a length-dependent, "stocking and glove" pattern.
- Because large myelinated sensory nerve fibers are primary players in proprioceptive pathways, testing frequently demonstrates diminished or lost joint position sense and ataxic gait. Assuming no motor neurons are affected, manual motor testing will likely be normal. Reflexes frequently are diminished or absent, often in a length-dependent pattern.
- In patients with sensory neuronopathies, involvement of the DRG can lead to altered sensation in variable, patchy distributions throughout the arms, legs, and trunk, or patients may demonstrate generalized alteration of sensation. Patients will have evidence of severely impaired proprioception, which in the most extreme cases will result in involuntary writhing movements of the fingers and toes, a phenomenon called pseudoathetosis.
- With trigeminal ganglion involvement, altered sensation may be detected in any combination of the V1 and V2 divisions or the sensory component of V3.
- Saccadic pursuits or nystagmus, due to impaired proprioceptive signaling from the vestibular system or extraocular muscles, can occur in advanced cases.
- Assuming no motor neurons are affected, manual motor testing should reveal full strength, though sustained full effort may not be possible due to impaired position sense. Reflexes may be diminished or absent due to dysfunction of the afferent sensory arc.
- While the neurologic examination provides information for localization, extraneural manifestations provide additional clues to aid in diagnosis. Careful skin, musculoskeletal, head and neck, and pulmonary assessments are particularly important. Rashes or inflamed joints often indicate an infectious or immune-mediated etiology. A rash in a dermatomal distribution may signify acute herpes zoster. Dry mucus membranes, a clinical hallmark of Sjögren syndrome, may point to an immunologic cause. Systemic changes such as weight loss and involvement of other organ

systems, particularly the pulmonary, gastrointestinal, and reproductive systems, are concerning for malignancy and associated paraneoplastic disorders.

Electrodiagnostic Studies

Nerve conduction testing and electromyography further assist in diagnosis by demonstrating the pattern and type of nerve involvement. Nerve conduction studies are normal in small fiber neuropathies. A normal study can be very helpful in supporting a diagnosis of small fiber neuropathy in a patient with a classic history and exam.

- Nerve conduction testing in large fiber sensory neuropathies usually demonstrates reduced or absent sensory nerve action potential (SNAP) amplitudes in a length-dependent pattern. Depending on the cause of neuropathy, demyelinating changes, with slowed conduction velocities and prolonged peak latencies, or axonal changes, with reduced SNAP amplitudes, are seen. Compound muscle action potentials (CMAPs) are normal assuming no motor involvement, though many large fiber sensory neuropathies can progress to have a motor component with resultant axonal or demyelinating changes.

In sensory neuronopathies, the nerve conduction studies demonstrate profoundly reduced or absent SNAP amplitudes in a generalized or multifocal pattern rather than a length-dependent pattern. When upper extremity SNAPs are more severely affected than lower extremity SNAPs, this is highly suggestive of localization to the DRG. Compound muscle action potentials are normal in pure sensory neuronopathies, though slowed conduction velocity and some reduction in CMAP amplitudes can be seen in various types. Blink reflex studies are useful when evaluating involvement of trigeminal nerve fibers and ganglia and may help differentiate Sjögren syndrome and idiopathic sensory neuronopathies, in which they will be abnormal, from paraneoplastic sensory neuronopathies, in which they should be normal. Electromyography often is normal, though patients may struggle with activation due to impaired proprioceptive input and denervation of muscle spindles and Golgi tendon organs. Mildly increased insertional and abnormal spontaneous activity with subtle chronic neurogenic changes may be seen in certain cases.

Autonomic Studies

In small fiber neuropathies, especially those with clinical symptoms of dysautonomia, autonomic testing can be a useful diagnostic tool. The two tests that are most often utilized are the Quantitative Sudomotor Axon Reflex Test (QSART) and thermoregulatory sweat testing. QSART assesses sudomotor function by detecting sweat production after acetylcholine is iontophoresed into the skin. Sudomotor function is mediated by postganglionic unmyelinated sympathetic axons. Sweat response is measured from four standard sites: proximal foot, distal leg, proximal leg, and forearm. There is a correlation between QSART abnormalities and loss of intraepidermal nerve fibers on skin biopsy.

During thermoregulatory sweat testing, the patient's body temperature is raised in a hot, humid setting. The body is covered in an indicator dye that measures sweat production. Photographs of sweat distribution are used to calculate the percentage of anhidrosis. Thermoregulatory sweat testing and sudomotor testing have been reported to be abnormal in the clear majority of patients with small fiber neuropathy. Testing of cardiovagal function with the Valsalva ratio and heart rate response to deep breathing, and sympathetic adrenergic function with the beat-to-beat blood pressure response during Valsalva maneuver and head-up tilt, are typically low yield in small fiber neuropathies but may be abnormal in the sensory neuropathies with more profound autonomic dysfunction, such as in patients with paraneoplastic neuropathy and amyloidosis.

Laboratory Studies

The clinical history, physical examination, and electrodiagnostic findings can help to determine which laboratory studies will be most useful. These studies will vary depending on the localization, time course, and clinical context. As sensory neuropathies can be caused by numerous etiologies, it requires some restraint on the part of the physician to resist over-ordering studies with low diagnostic yield. Very broadly, sensory nerve diseases can be acquired, inherited, and idiopathic. Nearly 30% to 50% of patients with sensory neuropathy will ultimately be classified as having idiopathic conditions and, therefore, will have an unremarkable laboratory workup. The American Academy of Neurology and the American Association of Neuromuscular and Electrodiagnostic Medicine have both published evidence-based guidelines for the evaluation of distal symmetric polyneuropathies. Laboratory testing must be used judiciously and strongly influenced by the exam, electrodiagnostic studies, and clinical context, given the low etiologic yield of many studies.

- The laboratory studies with the highest diagnostic yield include blood glucose, serum vitamin B_{12}, and serum protein electrophoresis. The laboratory testing approach will be influenced by a number of factors, such as family history of neuropathy, exposure to a neurotoxic drug or excessive alcohol consumption, or history of HIV, as a few examples.
- Spinal fluid analysis and imaging studies are of relatively low yield in the sensory nerve diseases, with some specific exceptions. In the sensory forms of chronic inflammatory demyelinating polyradiculoneuropathy (CIDP), albuminocytological dissociation can be a supportive finding. In paraneoplastic sensory neuronopathies,

cerebrospinal fluid may have elevated protein, pleocytosis, and oligoclonal bands.

Imaging Studies

Imaging studies are mandatory in paraneoplastic neuropathies to look for an underlying malignancy. If routine radiographic studies are unremarkable, a fluorodeoxyglucose-positron emission tomography (FDG-PET) study is recommended, with surveillance imaging occurring every 6 months for up to 4 years after diagnosis. Neural axis and body imaging determines the extent of disease burden in patients with sarcoidosis and may identify a lymph node or other lesion for biopsy to confirm the diagnosis. Imaging of the spinal cord with MRI may demonstrate T_2 hyperintensity in the dorsal columns in Sjögren syndrome patients with sensory neuronopathy or in vitamin B_{12} or copper deficiency myeloneuropathies.

Tissue Biopsy

Skin

The skin biopsy is recommended by both American and European practice guidelines in the diagnosis of small fiber neuropathy and is considered the pathologic gold standard. The sensitivities and specificities of skin biopsies vary widely depending on the study, as the clinical standard has been used in their calculation. They can be easily performed by taking a 3-mm punch biopsy at the standard distance of 10 cm above the lateral malleolus at the distal leg. Biopsies of additional sites such as the distal and proximal thigh, foot, and upper extremity may be helpful in the setting of a non-length-dependent pattern.

Measurement of the intraepidermal nerve fiber density is the parameter most often used to determine the presence of a small fiber neuropathy. An antibody to protein gene product 9.5 is used to visualize and quantify the density of intraepidermal nerve fibers. Additionally, sudomotor fibers that innervate sweat glands and pilomotor fibers that innervate the arrector pilorum muscles can be studied to support autonomic nervous system involvement.

Nerve

Peripheral nerve and dorsal root ganglion biopsy adds very little to diagnostic evaluation of sensory predominant neuropathies. Peripheral sensory nerves, in general, are biopsied if there is a clinical suspicion of vasculitis, sarcoidosis, or lymphoma. Dorsal root ganglion biopsies, because of the risk of complication, are essentially contraindicated in the workup of sensory neuronopathies.

Other

Other tissues may need to be biopsied to support or confirm a specific sensory neuropathy diagnosis. The classic examples include biopsy of a tumor in a paraneoplastic neuropathy, a salivary gland biopsy in a patient with sicca symptoms to support a diagnosis of Sjögren syndrome, a lymph node biopsy in a patient with sarcoidosis, or an abdominal fat pad biopsy in a patient with suspected amyloidosis. These assessments are covered in more detail in the differential diagnosis section.

DIFFERENTIAL DIAGNOSIS

The differential diagnosis of the sensory nerve disorders can be considered in terms of localization (small fiber, large fiber, DRG, dorsal columns, and trigeminal nerve) as well as by category of etiology (metabolic, autoimmune, infectious, toxic, neoplastic, hereditary, and idiopathic).

Small Fiber Neuropathies

A review of the most common and important etiologies of small fiber neuropathies follows. For a comprehensive list of disorders and disease states associated with small fiber involvement, refer to Table 8.1. The standard rule that positive sensory symptoms imply an acquired cause whereas a painless neuropathy implies an inherited condition does not necessarily hold true in small fiber neuropathies. As an example, the small fiber neuropathies associated with Fabry disease and sodium channel mutations are quite painful. If an underlying etiology cannot be defined and the patient lacks a family history of neuropathy, the patient likely has an idiopathic small fiber neuropathy.

- Regarding metabolic etiologies, diabetes mellitus is the most common cause of peripheral neuropathy in the world and may cause a small fiber neuropathy, a large fiber sensory neuropathy, or a sensorimotor neuropathy, often with autonomic features. Glucose intolerance, as defined by a fasting glucose greater than or equal to 100 to 125 milligrams/deciliter (mg/dL), a 2-hour oral glucose tolerance test of 140 to 199 mg/dL, or a glycosylated hemoglobin between 5.7% and 6.4% is also associated with sensory neuropathy development. In patients who would otherwise be labeled as having idiopathic sensory neuropathy, nearly half have evidence of impaired glucose tolerance. It is debated whether this is an association or causative. Metabolic syndrome—which comprises the constellation of diabetes or impaired glucose tolerance, dyslipidemia, central obesity, and elevated blood pressure—is also associated with small fiber neuropathies. Hypertriglyceridemia in isolation may be an independent risk factor for developing small fiber neuropathy.

- Treatment-induced neuropathy diabetes, also known as "insulin neuritis," is an under-recognized cause of small fiber dysfunction in the setting of rapid correction of hyperglycemia. It has been

TABLE 8.1 Small Fiber Neuropathies

Etiology of small fiber neuropathy	Recommended investigations
Metabolic	
• Glucose dysglycemia	
▫ Diabetes mellitus	Hemoglobin A1c, fasting blood sugar, 2-hour oral glucose tolerance test
▫ Impaired fasting glucose	2-hour oral glucose tolerance test, fasting blood sugar, hemoglobin A1c
▫ Treatment-induced neuropathy in diabetes (insulin neuritis)	Clinical diagnosis in the context of rapid correction of hyperglycemia
• Hyperlipidemia (specifically hypertriglyceridemia)	Lipid panel including triglyceride levels
• Metabolic syndrome	Clinical diagnosis of impaired glucose tolerance or diabetes mellitus, dyslipidemia, central obesity, and elevated blood pressure
• Thyroid dysfunction	TSH, free T_4
• Chronic kidney disease	BUN, creatinine
• Vitamin deficiency (B_1, B_{12})	B_1, B_{12}, methylmalonic acid
Autoimmune	
• Sjögren syndrome	Anti-SSA, anti-SSB antibodies, Schirmer's test, Rose Bengal test, lip/salivary gland biopsy
• Systemic lupus erythematosus	ANA, anti-dsDNA antibody, anti-Smith antibody, complement levels, antiphospholipid antibodies, ESR, CRP
• Sarcoidosis	Serum angiotensin-converting enzyme, chest x-ray, biopsy of affected tissue
• Celiac disease	Anti-gliadin antibodies (endomysial and tissue transglutaminase antibodies)
• Other autoimmune	"Dysimmune" conditions may have elevated inflammatory markers, plus often early-onset, severe, generalized, refractory pain with response to immunotherapy Anti-sulfatide antibodies
Infectious	
• Human immunodeficiency virus/ acquired immunodeficiency syndrome	HIV viral load, CD4 count

(continued)

TABLE 8.1 Small Fiber Neuropathies (*continued*)

Etiology of small fiber neuropathy	Recommended investigations
• Hepatitis C	Hepatitis C virus antibody, hepatitis C PCR
• Cryoglobulinemia	Typically occurs with hepatitis C and mixed cryoglobulinemia; hepatitis C virus antibody, hepatitis C PCR, and cryoglobulins
• Chagas disease	Chagas antibodies with ELISA
• Leprosy	Serum antibodies to phenolic glycolipid-I, skin or nerve biopsy for acid-fast bacilli
Amyloidosis	
• Systemic	Serum protein electrophoresis, immunofixation, serum light chains, urine protein electrophoresis, fat pad biopsy, rectal mucosal biopsy, kidney biopsy, skin biopsy
• Familial	Genetic testing for transthyretin, gelsolin, and APOA1
Drugs and toxins	
• Alcohol, metronidazole, nitrofurantoin, linezolid, anti-TNF α inhibitors, thallium, statins, chemotherapeutic agents, antiretrovirals, flecainide	Temporal relation to the toxin use and duration of use
Neoplastic	
• Multiple myeloma, monoclonal gammopathies	Serum protein electrophoresis, immunofixation, serum light chains, urine protein electrophoresis, bone marrow biopsy
• Paraneoplastic (often small cell lung cancer)	Anti-Hu, anti-CV2/CRMP5 antibodies, chest x-ray, chest CT, PET scan
Hereditary	
• Sodium channelopathies (Nav 1.7, Nav 1.8)	Genetic testing for SCN9A, SCN10A mutations
• Hereditary sensory and autonomic neuropathy	Genetic testing (many genetic mutations described)
• Fabry disease	Alpha-galactosidase A mutation (enzyme assay to measure alpha galactosidase activity)
• Ehlers-Danlos syndrome (hypermobile type)	Clinical diagnosis, hypermobile joints, and hyperextensible skin

(*continued*)

TABLE 8.1 Small Fiber Neuropathies (*continued*)

Etiology of small fiber neuropathy	Recommended investigations
• Hemochromatosis	Serum ferritin
Other	
• Fibromyalgia	Clinical diagnosis
• Idiopathic	Diagnosis of exclusion

ANA, antinuclear antibody; APOA1, apolipoprotein 1; BUN, blood urea nitrogen; CRP, C-reactive protein; CT, computed tomography; dsDNA, double-stranded DNA; dsDNA, double-stranded DNA; ELISA, enzyme-linked immunosorbent assay; ESR, erythrocyte sedimentation rate; HIV, human immunodeficiency virus; PCR, polymerase chain reaction; PET, positron emission tomography; TSH, thyroid-stimulating hormone.

reported in the setting of insulin use, oral hypoglycemic use, and even weight loss. The acute onset of severe neuropathic pain occurs typically within 2 months of the hyperglycemia correction and may be in a length-dependent pattern or more generalized. The greater the correction of the glycosylated hemoglobin, the higher the likelihood of developing treatment-inducted neuropathy in diabetes. Although aggressive neuropathic pain control is initially necessary, the pain usually improves within 2 years.

- Autoimmune small fiber neuropathies are diverse. They may be associated with primary rheumatologic diseases such as Sjögren syndrome, or they may be seen in other systemic autoimmune diseases such as sarcoidosis and celiac disease (CD). Sjögren syndrome is strongly associated with a wide array of neuropathies, including small fiber neuropathy, large fiber sensory neuropathy, sensorimotor neuropathy, and sensory neuronopathy. Sjögren syndrome–associated small fiber neuropathy is often multifocal and patchy, characterized by autonomic dysfunction, and has trigeminal nerve involvement. The peripheral neuropathy may be the initial manifestation of Sjögren syndrome and sicca symptoms may be absent. Additionally, Sjögren-specific antibodies (anti-SSA and anti-SSB) may be absent in up to 50% of patients with Sjögren syndrome neuropathy. As a consequence, reliance on additional diagnostic techniques such as Schirmer's testing, Rose Bengal testing, and lip or salivary gland biopsy may be necessary.

- In sarcoidosis, small fiber neuropathy is present in up to 40% of patients. The neuropathy pattern is length-dependent or non-length-dependent, and autonomic dysfunction is often present. As the small fiber symptoms are disabling despite good disease control, sarcoidosis is thought to be cytokine mediated, rather than the result of granulomatous infiltration.

- CD is an immune-mediated enteropathy that occurs in individuals with sensitivity to gluten. Patients will have symptoms of chronic malabsorptive diarrhea, flatulence, and weight loss. Distal symmetric sensory-predominant neuropathy is the most common subtype of neuropathy associated with CD. The prevalence of strictly small fiber polyneuropathy in patients with CD is unknown. Anti-TTG-IgA antibody markers have been identified in 3.5% of patients with otherwise idiopathic small fiber polyneuropathy. CD also causes ataxia and large fiber neuropathy.

- Emerging evidence indicates that some forms of idiopathic small fiber polyneuropathy are due to acute or chronic tissue-specific dysimmunity. A series of patients with early-onset small fiber neuropathy and refractory pain has been reported. In this series, 89% of the patients were noted to have serologic markers of disordered immunity. In support of the autoimmune pathophysiology, many patients benefited from immunomodulatory therapy. Therefore immunomodulatory (e.g., intravenous immune globulins [IVIG]) or immunosuppressant (e.g., prednisone) medications should be considered in patients with early-onset, intractable small fiber neuropathy without an identifiable etiology.

- Fibromyalgia is a heterogeneous disease characterized by widespread pain and fatigue. Recent studies have reported an association between fibromyalgia and small fiber neuropathy, confirmed by decreased intraepidermal nerve fiber density on skin biopsy.

- A common etiology of toxic small fiber neuropathies is ethanol. These neuropathies result from dysfunction of the small thinly myelinated and unmyelinated nerve fibers early on. They represent a separate type of neuropathy from thiamine-associated neuropathy, which is motor predominant and improves with thiamine repletion.

- Amyloidosis, both acquired light chain (AL) amyloidosis and familial amyloid polyneuropathy, causes small fiber neuropathy usually associated with autonomic dysfunction. Light chain amyloidosis is a plasma cell disorder in which monoclonal immunoglobulin light chains accumulate in tissues including the heart, kidneys, liver, and peripheral and autonomic nervous systems. Small fiber involvement manifesting as painful dysesthesia is an early symptom. The small fiber neuropathy typically progresses to a sensorimotor neuropathy, although other variable presentations such as multifocal mononeuropathies, plexopathies, and a CIDP-like presentation have been reported.

- Familial amyloid polyneuropathy is a group of autosomal dominant disorders characterized by cardiomyopathy and nephropathy in addition to progressive neuropathy. Common genetic mutations include transthyretin, apolipoprotein A1, and gelsolin. Transthyretin familial amyloidosis, the best described variant, is common in Portugal, Japan, and Sweden. The Val30Met substitution is the most prevalent genotype.

- Fabry disease is an X-linked disease due to a mutation in the *GLA* gene that leads to a deficiency of the alpha-galactosidase A enzyme. This lysosomal storage disorder results from accumulation of globotriaosylceramide in various organs, including the kidney, heart, central, and peripheral nervous systems. Patients often have angiokeratomas (dark red spots on the skin) and corneal opacities. From a neurologic perspective, Fabry disease presents with cerebrovascular disease, small fiber neuropathy, and dysautonomia.

- The hereditary sensory and autonomic neuropathies (HSANs) are a category of inherited neuropathies, some of which are dominantly inherited and some of which are recessively inherited. Many of them lead to small fiber dysfunction early on with neuropathic pain, but then go on to have large fiber and motor involvement as well as acromutilation.

- Mutations of voltage-gated sodium channels Nav 1.7 and Nav 1.8 may cause inherited, painful small fiber neuropathies and erythromelalgia. Dominant gain-of-function mutations of the *SCN9A* and *SCN10A* genes that encode Nav 1.7 and Nav 1.8, respectively, cause the syndrome. Nav 1.7 and Nav 1.8 are preferentially expressed in the small DRG neurons and cutaneous afferents. Nav 1.7 is expressed in peripheral sensory and visceral sensory neurons.

Large Fiber Neuropathies

In this section, the common forms of large fiber sensory neuropathies with a length-dependent pattern are discussed. As mentioned, many of these neuropathies fall within a spectrum; that is, they may initially have significant small fiber nerve dysfunction and evolve over time to affect the larger nerve fibers as well. Only the neuropathies most classically associated with large fiber dysfunction are reviewed here. For a diagnostic and treatment algorithm for patients with acquired, axonal, large fiber sensory-predominant neuropathies, refer to Figure 8.1.

- Diabetes is the most common cause of all neuropathies, large fiber neuropathies included.

- Hypothyroidism also causes a neuropathy with both small and large fiber-mediated symptoms and deficits on exam.

- Other metabolic etiologies of primarily sensory neuropathies are caused by nutritional deficiencies. Symptom onset for nutritional deficiencies is usually subacute to chronic, and most patients present with a length-dependent pattern of sensory loss.
  - Vitamin B_{12} and copper deficiencies cause a myeloneuropathy, such that patients may have upper motor neuron signs on exam. Vitamin B_{12} deficiency may present with non-length-dependent sensory loss as well and should be considered especially in the context of malnutrition and malabsorption.

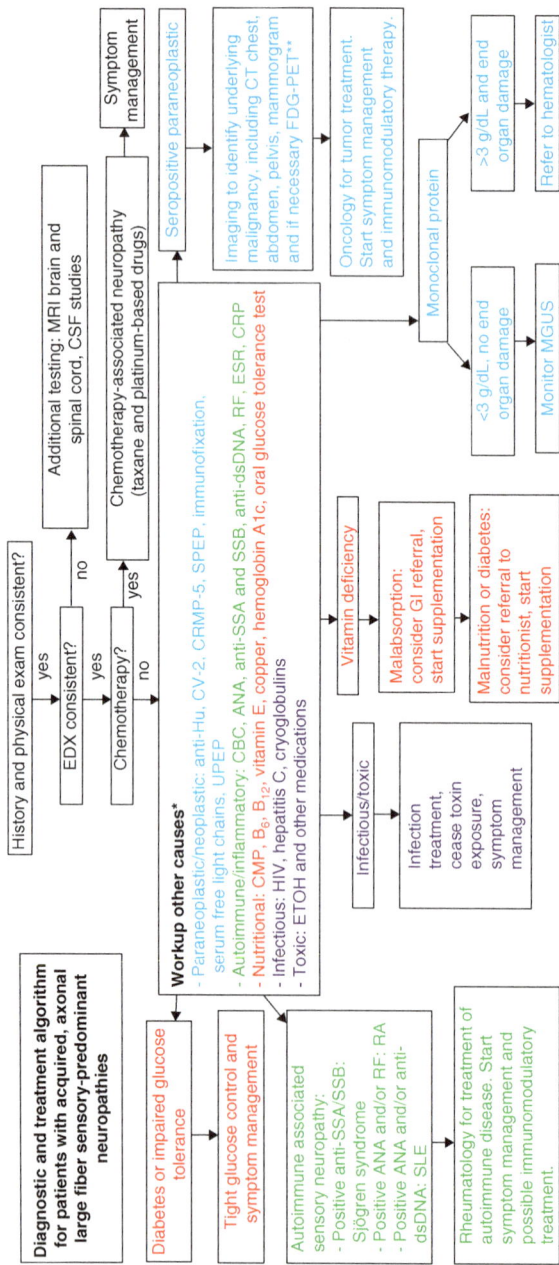

FIGURE 8.1 Diagnostic and treatment algorithm for patients with acquired, axonal large fiber sensory predominant neuropathies.

*This is a list of the more common laboratory investigations for large fiber sensory neuropathies. The studies should be ordered based on clinical context and index of suspicion.

** Imaging for an underlying malignancy in seropositive paraneoplastic syndrome includes surveillance imaging every 6 months for up to 4 years.

ANA, antinuclear antibody; CBC, complete blood count; CMP, comprehensive metabolic panel; CRP, C-reactive protein; CSF, cerebrospinal fluid; CT, computed tomography; dsDNA, double-stranded DNA; EDX, electrodiagnostic testing; ESR, erythrocyte sedimentation rate; FDG-PET, fluorodeoxyglucose-positron emission tomography; GI, gastrointestinal; HIV, human immunodeficiency virus; MGUS, monoclonal gammopathy of undetermined significance; RF, rheumatoid factor; SLE, systemic lupus erythematosus; SPEP, serum protein electrophoresis; UPEP, urine protein electrophoresis.

- Vitamin E deficiency leads to large fiber sensory loss, resulting in profound ataxia, and should be considered in the differential diagnosis of patients presenting with early-onset ataxia.
- Thiamine (or vitamin B_1) deficiency causes an axonal sensorimotor polyneuropathy. It has also been reported to mimic Guillain-Barré syndrome with an acute, motor-predominant presentation.
- Vitamin B_6 deficiency associated with neuropathy has most often been described in the context of isoniazid use in patients with tuberculosis. Otherwise, the role of vitamin B_6 deficiency in neuropathy is rather unclear, and supplementation of vitamin B_6 in other forms of neuropathy appears to be futile. Folic acid deficiency has been reported to cause a slowly progressive, symmetric, distal, sensory-predominant axonal large fiber neuropathy. Table 8.2 lists nutritional deficiency-associated neuropathies and their treatments.
- There are many other autoimmune causes of sensory large fiber neuropathy, apart from those associated with classic rheumatological conditions. An entire category of autoimmune sensory-predominant neuropathies present with early-onset ataxia and pathology localizing to the nerve roots and peripheral nerves (as opposed to the DRG). These are helpful to consider in the context of pace of symptom onset, differentiating those with an acute presentation from those with a more chronic, indolent course, and in the context of localization either to the axons or to the peripheral myelin. For a list of neuropathies that present with early-onset ataxia, refer to Table 8.3.
- Acute ataxic neuropathies include Miller Fisher syndrome, which presents as ophthalmoplegia, ataxia, and areflexia often following an antecedent infection, with *Campylobacter jejuni* being the most reported infectious organism. Most patients with Miller Fisher syndrome will have antibodies that react with the disialosyl ganglioside GQ1b. On nerve conduction studies, there is evidence of a peripheral sensory axonal neuropathy. Many patients experience a rapid reversibility of the sensory electrophysiological abnormalities, suggesting dysfunction of the nodal and paranodal regions. Patients with slow improvement may have axonal degeneration. Some patients without ophthalmoplegia may be better classified as "ataxic Guillain-Barré syndrome."
- Acute sensory ataxic neuropathy (ASAN) is associated with antibodies to GD1b and other disialosyl gangliosides. These patients have an acute, monophasic illness characterized by ataxia and sensory signs. It is hypothesized that this condition is due to dysfunction of the nodes of Ranvier of the sensory axons given patients' rapid recovery. This condition has significant clinical

TABLE 8.2 Neuropathies Associated With Vitamin Deficiencies

Nutrient	Presentation	Confirmatory testing	Treatment recommendations
Vitamin B_{12} deficiency	Myeloneuropathy	Serum vitamin B_{12} and methylmalonic acid. Consider gastrin and intrinsic factor antibodies if concerned for pernicious anemia.	1 mg intramuscular or subcutaneous weekly for 1 month; then monthly thereafter unless a reversible cause is found
Folic acid	Sensory neuropathy	Serum folic acid	1 mg/day
Copper deficiency	Myeloneuropathy	Serum copper Consider zinc toxicity	Elemental copper: 8 mg daily orally for 1 week, then decrease by 2 mg every week and continue 2 mg daily thereafter unless a reversible cause is found
Vitamin E deficiency	Sensory neuropathy with prominent ataxia and cerebellar features	Serum vitamin E	50 to 200 IU orally daily unless a reversible cause is found
Vitamin B_1 (thiamine) deficiency	Motor predominant sensorimotor polyneuropathy	Serum vitamin B_1	100 mg IV or IM for 3–5 days, followed by 50 mg orally daily
Vitamin B_6 (pyridoxine) deficiency or toxicity	Deficiency: length-dependent neuropathy Toxicity: sensory neuronopathy	Serum vitamin B_6	Deficiency: 50 mg daily orally in patients taking isoniazid or long-term hydralazine treatment Toxicity: stop vitamin B_6 supplementation

IM, intramuscular; IV, intravenous.

overlap with ataxic Guillain-Barré syndrome and is likely part of the same clinical spectrum.

- Chronic ataxic neuropathy with disialosyl antibodies (CANDA) is characterized by marked sensory ataxia with relatively preserved motor function in the limbs. Patients have IgM antibodies that

TABLE 8.3 Ataxic Neuropathies

Etiology	Associated features and comments
Autoimmune	
• Miller Fisher syndrome	• Antecedent infection, often *Campylobacter jejuni* • Ophthalmoparesis, ataxia, areflexia • Anti-GQ1b antibody
• Acute sensory ataxic neuropathy	• Overlap with ataxic Guillain-Barré syndrome • Anti-GD1b antibody
• GALOP syndrome	• Gait disorder (early-onset ataxia) • Autoantibody to central myelin antigen • Late-age onset • Polyneuropathy • Associated with IgM monoclonal protein
• Anti-MAG antibody syndrome (distal acquired demyelinating syndrome [DADS])	• IgM monoclonal protein • Often in older men • MAG antibody is present • Polyneuropathy with distal demyelination
• Chronic immune sensory polyradiculoneuropathy (CISP)	• Normal nerve conduction studies • Abnormal somatosensory evoked potentials
• CANOMAD	• Chronic ataxic neuropathy • Ophthalmoplegia • IgM monoclonal protein • Cold agglutinins • Disialosyl antibodies
Sensory neuronopathy	
• Anti-Hu, anti-CV2/CRMP-5	Paraneoplastic associated often with small cell lung cancer
• Sjögren syndrome	Anti-SSA, anti-SSB antibodies, sicca symptoms
• Idiopathic	
Toxic	
• Vitamin B₆ toxicity	• Sensory neuronopathy • Seen with doses as little as 200 mg/day
• Cis-platinum	• Sensory neuropathy/neuronopathy
Infectious	
• Syphilis (tabes dorsalis)	• Dorsal column dysfunction, autonomic dysfunction, Argyll Robertson pupil, aortitis, MHA-TP, VDRL

(continued)

TABLE 8.3 Ataxic Neuropathies (*continued*)

Etiology	Associated features and comments
Nutritional deficiency	
• Vitamin B$_{12}$	• Dorsal column and peripheral neuropathy affecting large fibers • Distal weakness • Hyporeflexia or hyperreflexia • Autonomic dysfunction • Megaloblastic anemia
• Vitamin E	• Seen with malabsorption • Ataxic polyneuropathy with cerebellar features • Ophthalmoplegia

IgM, immunoglobulin M; MHA-TP, microhemagglutination assay for treponemal antibodies; VDRL, Venereal Disease Research Laboratory.

react with disialosyl epitopes. When the full clinical syndrome is present, it goes by the acronym CANOMAD: chronic ataxic neuropathy, ophthalmoplegia, IgM paraprotein, cold agglutinins, and disialosyl antibodies. CANDA may be a less restrictive term given that many patients do not develop ophthalmoplegia. There is evidence of a sensory axonal neuropathy on nerve conduction studies, with variable motor conduction abnormalities.

- The chronic autoimmune demyelinating neuropathies with prominent sensory symptoms include the sensory variant of CIDP. Patients will have distal predominant pan-sensory or small fiber-predominant sensory impairment, pain, and paresthesia. Motor involvement is absent or minimal. Dramatic ataxia is present in many patients. Despite the presence of marked sensory symptoms and signs, there is typically evidence of both motor and sensory demyelination on electrophysiological studies.

- Chronic immune sensory polyradiculoneuropathy (CISP) should be considered in patients with marked gait ataxia, impaired proprioception, and paresthesia. The patient's strength is entirely spared. Often standard electrophysiological studies are normal, whereas somatosensory evoked potentials are abnormal, supporting localization to the proximal roots. Cerebrospinal fluid protein is elevated and MRI may demonstrate enlarged lumbar roots. Patients often respond to treatment with IVIG and prednisone. This syndrome is often monophasic and treatment can ultimately be discontinued.

- Distal acquired demyelinating symmetric neuropathy (DADS) is an MAG-antibody–positive demyelinating neuropathy that presents with significant sensory loss affecting the distal extremities and the legs more so than the arms. It is classically a disease of older men. Patients present with early gait ataxia and, to a lesser extent, distal leg weakness. This slowly progressive neuropathy demonstrates distal demyelination on electrophysiological studies with markedly prolonged distal latencies, slowing of conduction velocities, and absent conduction block. Almost universally patients will have an IgM monoclonal protein, and MAG antibodies typify the disease. Treatments for CIDP such as IVIG and prednisone are not beneficial in DADS, whereas some patients may respond to rituximab, cyclophosphamide, and plasma exchange.

- Patients with antisulfatide antibody neuropathy often have distal sensory symptoms, and a minority will have weakness. The patterns of antisulfatide neuropathy may take many forms, including small fiber neuropathy, mixed large and small fiber sensory neuropathy, sensorimotor neuropathy, and demyelinating sensorimotor polyneuropathy.

- GALOP (gait disorder, autoantibody, late-age onset, polyneuropathy) is another later-onset polyneuropathy with early-onset ataxia and sensory predominant symptoms. Most patients will have an IgM monoclonal protein and may have an antibody to central myelin antigen. Treatment with cyclophosphamide and IVIG may be beneficial.

- Infectious causes of large fiber sensory neuropathies are diverse. Hepatitis C and associated cryoglobulinemia cause a neuropathy that classically presents in a pain-predominant, mononeuropathy multiplex pattern, due to necrotizing vasculitis of the sensory nerves primarily. Notably, this is one of the few sensory neuropathies that, as opposed to neuronopathies, presents in a non-length-dependent, asymmetrical fashion.

- Chronic hepatitis B, in the absence of an association with polyarteritis nodosa, is loosely associated with sensorimotor polyneuropathies. The neuropathy associated with polyarteritis nodosa is mostly vasculitic and, therefore, has a significant motor component; it is not discussed further here.

- HIV can present in a multitude of ways, affecting the autonomic, motor, and sensory systems. The most common pattern of sensory nerve involvement is a distal, symmetric, painful neuropathy. This pathology is thought to be due to axonal degeneration affecting the distal regions of the body, loss of unmyelinated fibers, and macrophage infiltration into the peripheral nerves and DRG. The predominant feature is pain, and onset is gradual. Feet may become very tender, such that donning socks and shoes becomes quite painful, and patients can develop an antalgic gait pattern. Symptoms may slowly ascend over several months and, upon reaching knee level, may start to involve the fingertips as well.

- Toxic causes of large fiber sensory neuropathies may present more subacutely to acutely and are typically length dependent.

However, with certain topical industrial chemical exposures (e.g., acrylide monomer), nerve damage will occur at and distal to the site of exposure. Thankfully, occupational exposures to industrial toxins are uncommon in developed countries, though certain inhalants, particularly hexacarbons, are used recreationally and can lead to neuropathy. Numerous medications outlined in Table 8.4 can also cause peripheral nerve dysfunction.

- Paraproteinemic neuropathies, ranging from monoclonal gammopathies of undetermined significance (MGUS), which is the

TABLE 8.4 Toxic Neuropathies

Medication class: name	Presentation
Anesthetic: nitrous oxide	Myeloneuropathy due to vitamin B_{12} deficiency from irreversible oxidization of cobalamin
Antigout: colchicine	Length-dependent, sensory-predominant, axonal neuropathy (may occur in combination with a myopathy)
Antihypertensive: hydralazine (only with long-term, high doses)	Length-dependent, sensory-predominant, axonal neuropathy
Antimicrobial: chloramphenicol, ethambutol, metronidazole	Length-dependent, sensory-predominant, axonal neuropathy Chloramphenicol often causes a more pain-predominant presentation
Antineoplastic: platinum-based chemotherapy, taxanes, vinca alkaloids, etoposide and teniposide, epothilones, ado-trastuzumab emtansine, bortezomib, ifosfamide, proteasome inhibitors (less common)	Length-dependent, often painful, sensorimotor, axonal neuropathy
Antiepileptic: phenytoin	Length-dependent, sensorimotor, axonal neuropathy
Antitubercular: isoniazid	Length-dependent, sensory-predominant, axonal neuropathy
Immunosuppressant: leflunomide, thalidomide	Length-dependent, painful, sensory-predominant, axonal neuropathy
Nucleoside analogue reverse transcriptase inhibitors: zalcitabine (ddC), stavudine (d4T), didanosine (ddI)	Length-dependent, painful, sensory-predominant, axonal neuropathy
Pyridoxine excess	Sensory neuronopathy

most common, to amyloidosis and multiple myeloma, are due to the clonal proliferation of B lymphocytes or plasma cells. There are four clinical paraproteinemic neuropathy subtypes: CIDP, a distal demyelinating neuropathy (DADS), small fiber neuropathy with prominent autonomic features, and axonal sensorimotor neuropathy. These diseases can present subacutely or in a more indolent fashion, often with multisystem involvement, particularly affecting the heart, kidneys, and skeletal system. Amyloidosis has been covered more extensively under small fiber neuropathies. A minority of patients with multiple myeloma will have a length-dependent sensory predominant neuropathy prior to undergoing treatment.

- Paraneoplastic neurologic syndromes are diverse. Both anti-Hu and anti-CRMP-5/CV2 mediated paraneoplastic neuropathies are associated with small fiber neuropathies, sensorimotor neuropathies, and sensory neuronopathies. Anti-Hu and anti-CRMP-5/CV2 are covered in more detail in the sensory neuronopathy section. Separately, the autoantibodies targeting the neuronal voltage-gated potassium-channel complex results in a spectrum of peripheral nervous system manifestations including a chronic pain syndrome and a length-dependent, sensory-predominant, axonal neuropathy. The voltage-gated potassium-channel complex targets leucine-rich glioma-inactivated 1 (LGI1) and contactin-associated protein 2 (CASPR2). Patients with the peripheral nervous system manifestations are most likely to have CASPR2 antibodies. Those patients with chronic pain will often have a normal electrophysiological study, but show evidence of neuronal hyperexcitability including hyperhidrosis and quantitative heat-pain hyperalgesia. Several patients with CASPR2 who experienced refractory pain or sensory neuropathy have derived significant benefits from immunotherapy.

- Chronic idiopathic axonal polyneuropathy is one of the most common types of neuropathies. It is a slowly progressive, sensory or sensorimotor axonal neuropathy. It starts on average in the sixth decade of life and is slightly more prevalent in males. It is a diagnosis of exclusion.

Dorsal Root Ganglia

Dysfunction of the DRG may be a localized process, such as in herpes zoster, or a more generalized condition, such as in paraneoplastic sensory neuronopathy. The presentation and differential diagnoses are dissimilar.

- If a patient presents with a vesicular rash following a dermatomal pattern (shingles) or history of these symptoms plus positive neuropathic symptoms following a similar distribution, varicella zoster virus (VZV) should be high on the differential diagnosis list. VZV infiltrates sensory ganglia and establishes latency, with intermittent reactivation, over the lifetime of the host. Once the VZV is reactivated, there is an intense inflammatory response in the DRG. Postherpetic neuralgia, defined as the persistence of pain for greater than 3 months after rash has healed, is a common complication of VZV infections. Symptoms are typically unilateral and restricted to a specific dermatome, though systemic infections, particularly in immunocompromised patients, are possible. The diagnosis is more challenging when the patient develops a dermatomal band of numbness and pain in the absence of a rash. The differential diagnosis in this case would include Lyme neuroborreliosis resulting in a painful radiculopathy and diabetic thoracic radiculopathy, which often has motor involvement manifesting as abdominal wall weakness.

- Though these conditions are rare, the causes of sensory neuronopathies are diverse. Figure 8.2 provides a diagnostic and treatment algorithm for them. By far the most common autoimmune cause of sensory neuronopathy is Sjögren syndrome. Sicca symptoms (xerophthalmia and xerostomia) are the clinical hallmark of this disease, although the peripheral nervous system manifestations may predate these. Symptom onset is subacute, taking weeks to months to manifest fully, and the mean age of onset of Sjögren-associated sensory neuronopathy is 65. Forty percent of all peripheral neuropathies associated with Sjögren syndrome are sensory neuronopathies. Other presentations discussed elsewhere in this chapter include small and large fiber neuropathies. Sensorimotor neuropathy, vasculitic neuropathy, polyradiculopathy, dysautonomia, and cranial neuropathies also can occur. Lastly, common extraneural pathologies include myopathy, renal tubular acidosis, bronchiolitis, and pancreatitis.

- Celiac disease is a chronic autoimmune disorder causing severe adverse reactions to gluten protein, including scarring of the intestinal lining. Patients may report severe abdominal cramping, diarrhea, and even bloody stools after gluten ingestion. Central and peripheral nervous system involvement occurs in nearly 30% of patients. The link between sensory neuronopathy and CD is disputed, as many of the reported patients have had an alternative diagnosis to explain their neuropathy and many of those reported in the literature to have CD-associated sensory neuronopathy did not have enteropathy on biopsy. There have been case reports of other autoimmune causes of this sensory neuronopathy, including autoimmune hepatitis and systemic lupus erythematosus.

- Certain medications and supplements are known to cause sensory neuronopathies.

  - Vitamin B_6, essential to amino acid metabolism, can be toxic in excess. Toxicity is dose dependent, such that some patients

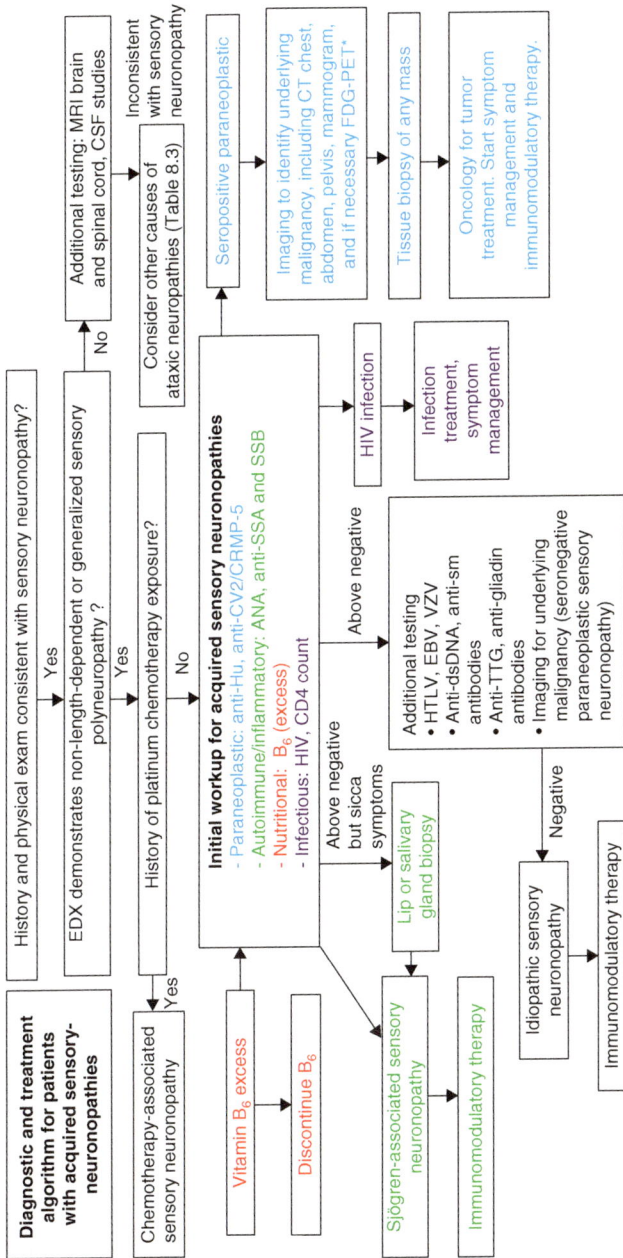

FIGURE 8.2 Diagnostic and treatment algorithm for patients with acquired sensory neuronopathies.

* Imaging for an underlying malignancy in seropositive paraneoplastic syndrome includes surveillance imaging every 6 months for up to 4 years.

ANA, antinuclear antibody; dsDNA, double-stranded DNA; EBV, Epstein-Barr virus; EDX, electrodiagnostic testing; FDG-PET, fluorodeoxyglucose-positron emission tomography; HIV, human immunodeficiency virus; HTLV, human T-lymphotropic virus; sm, Smith; TTG, tissue transglutaminase; VZV, varicella zoster virus.

taking as little as 200 mg/day may develop sensory neuronopathies. Because of this dose dependence, chronic exposure is needed to reach toxic levels, and patients may not become symptomatic until after they have maintained supplementation for many months. This diagnosis can be elicited based on patient history with careful review of medications and elevated vitamin B_6 serum concentrations.

- Chemotherapeutic agents, platinum-based drugs (cisplatin, carboplatin, and oxaliplatin) can induce apoptosis of the DRG sensory neurons in a dose-dependent fashion. A cumulative dose of 300 milligrams/meter^2 (mg/m^2) of cisplatin can cause positive neuropathic symptoms. Nearly all patients who receive more than 400 to 500 mg/m^2 experience peripheral neurotoxicity after 3 to 6 months of treatment. Sometimes patients can develop symptoms several months after completing chemotherapy treatments—a phenomenon known as the "coasting effect." Though carboplatin is not as neurotoxic as cisplatin and oxaliplatin, when it is combined with paclitaxel a severe sensory neuronopathy can result. Diagnosis of chemotherapy-induced sensory neuronopathy can be elucidated based upon history, electrodiagnostic findings, and physical exam findings.

- When a patient presents with unexplained weight loss, possible systemic involvement, and subacute onset of sensory neuronopathy symptoms, paraneoplastic etiology should be high on the differential diagnosis list. Anti-Hu antibodies are the antibody type most commonly linked to paraneoplastic sensory neuronopathy, though anti-CRMP5/CV2 antibodies have also been reported. Patients present with subacute-onset sensory ataxia; some may experience painful neuropathic symptoms as well. Patients may also have motor nerve, cerebellar, brainstem, or neuromuscular junction involvement in the form of Lambert-Eaton myasthenic syndrome. Autonomic dysfunction is not uncommon. Patients may present with tonic pupils, orthostasis, gastroparesis, and sicca symptoms. Anti-Hu antibodies are strongly predictive of underlying malignancy and may precede cancer diagnosis by anywhere from 3 to 8 months. The most commonly associated cancer is small cell lung cancer, but breast cancer, ovarian cancer, Hodgkin lymphoma, urologic tumors, and neuroendocrine tumors have been linked to this condition as well.

- Hereditary and degenerative causes of sensory neuronopathy are rare, present differently than the acquired causes, and typically have significant motor involvement. Of these, Charcot-Marie-Tooth disease type 2B (CMT2B) is encountered more frequently and should be considered in the differential diagnosis if the patient's symptoms are consistent and there is a positive family history, although de novo mutations do occur. Charcot-Marie-Tooth disease type 2B, which is dominantly inherited, usually presents in the second or third decade of life. Weakness and numbness are symmetrical and prominent distally to a greater degree in the lower extremities. Patients typically have foot deformities (pes cavus and hammer toes) and can develop foot ulcers that can be painful and become infected. Autonomic dysfunction also can occur.

- If a thorough diagnostic evaluation reveals no known cause for the patient's sensory neuronopathy, the condition is considered idiopathic. This is the case for nearly half of all sensory neuronopathies and is a diagnosis of exclusion. Patients who fall into this category have a chronic, gradual onset of symptoms with a slowly progressive course. It is hypothesized that the idiopathic sensory neuronopathies are also autoimmune in nature.

Trigeminal Nerve

Trigeminal neuralgia (historically called "tic douloureux") is more common in women than in men, and idiopathic cases are more common after age 50. Most cases of "classic" trigeminal neuralgia are due to compression of the trigeminal nerve by an aberrant loop of an artery or vein. Trigeminal neuralgia has also been described in the context of structural lesions such as vestibular schwannomas, meningiomas, aneurysms, and other vascular malformations. In the differential diagnosis of trigeminal neuralgia are short-lasting unilateral neuralgiform headache attacks (SUNHA). These headaches are characterized by conjunctival injection and tearing, unlike trigeminal neuralgia, and are included among the trigeminal autonomic cephalalgias.

In contrast to patients with trigeminal neuralgia, patients with trigeminal neuropathy may present with facial numbness in a trigeminal nerve distribution with variable degrees of weakness of the muscles of mastication. Trigeminal neuropathies may present with or without pain. The differential diagnosis list for these neuropathies is broad and includes metabolic causes such as diabetes, toxic causes such as specific drugs (e.g., oxaliplatin), autoimmune causes (mixed and undifferentiated connective tissue disease, scleroderma, Sjögren syndrome, sarcoidosis), infectious causes (VZV, herpes simplex virus, Lyme disease, leprosy), neoplastic causes (metastasis from breast or lung carcinoma; carcinomatous meningitis; compression from meningioma, trigeminal, or vestibular schwannoma), trauma to the nerve (surgical or dental procedure), pontomedullary ischemia or hemorrhage, vascular malformation, and idiopathic causes.

TREATMENT

The treatment of sensory nerve diseases consists of both symptomatic management of neuropathic pain and disease-specific management when appropriate.

Symptomatic Management of Neuropathic Pain

Most neuropathic pain medication trials have been conducted in the postherpetic neuralgia and painful diabetic neuropathy populations.

Oral treatment of neuropathic pain falls primarily in two categories: antidepressant and antiepileptic drugs. A few topical ointments and patches are available as well. Based on GRADE (Grading of Recommendations Assessment, Development, and Evaluation) recommendations, the first-line drugs for neuropathic pain include serotonin–norepinephrine reuptake inhibitors (duloxetine and venlafaxine), tricyclic antidepressants, and pregabalin, gabapentin, or gabapentin extended release. Second-line drugs include tramadol, capsaicin 8% patches and lidocaine patches. Third-line drugs are strong opioids and botulinum toxin A. Table 8.5 enumerates the medications most often used for neuropathic pain.

- Tricyclic antidepressants have analgesic properties mediated by inhibition of serotonin and norepinephrine reuptake, N-methyl-D-aspartate (NMDA), 5-HT, histamine, and muscarinic and α-adrenergic receptor antagonism. Sodium-channel inhibition occurs with some agents. Tricyclic antidepressants are considered a first choice by many clinicians because of their low cost and once-daily dosing. The side effects that are most commonly encountered relate to the drugs' anticholinergic properties. As such, patients may develop dry mouth, blurred vision, urinary retention, constipation, orthostatic hypotension, drowsiness, and weight gain. Tricyclic antidepressants may also cause confusion in the elderly. Nortriptyline is reported to have fewer anticholinergic side effects and causes less sedation. Tricyclic antidepressants are dosed at bedtime due to their sedative effects. A low dose should be started and gradually increased until the maximum benefit is appreciated.

- Serotonin–norepinephrine reuptake inhibitors include duloxetine and venlafaxine. Newer drugs in this category include desvenlafaxine, milnacipran, and levomilnacipran, which are not yet commonly used for neuropathic pain. Duloxetine may cause nausea, dry mouth, constipation, diarrhea, sedation, and dizziness. It is contraindicated in patients with severe hepatic dysfunction and uncontrolled hypertension. Venlafaxine is available in immediate-release and extended-release formulations; gastrointestinal side effects are the most common side effects with this drug. In a minority of patients elevated blood pressure may occur. Venlafaxine often needs to be titrated to doses on the high end of the dosing spectrum (150 mg/day to 225 mg/day) for neuropathic pain relief.

- The calcium-channel α-2-delta ligands, gabapentin and pregabalin, share a similar structure with gamma-aminobutyric acid (GABA) but do not bind GABA receptors. They work through binding to

TABLE 8.5 Common Neuropathic Pain Medications

Drug	Mechanism of action	Side effects	Dosing range	Precautions
Tricyclic antidepressants • Amitriptyline • Nortriptyline • Desipramine	Serotonin and norepinephrine reuptake inhibitors; block sodium channels and have anticholinergic properties	Anticholinergic effects (dry eyes/dry mouth, orthostatic hypotension, urinary retention), somnolence, weight gain	25–150 mg nightly	Use with caution in patients with cardiac disease and conduction abnormalities
Serotonin–norepinephrine reuptake inhibitors • Venlafaxine • Duloxetine	Inhibit reuptake of serotonin and norepinephrine	Nausea, hypertension, headache, sleep disturbance	Venlafaxine: Doses as high as 150–225 mg/day, divided twice daily, are often needed; extended-release formulation available Duloxetine: 60–120 mg/day May be divided into twice-daily dosing for doses greater than 60 mg/day	Venlafaxine: Use with caution in patients with cardiac disease, as it may cause tachycardia and hypertension Venlafaxine and duloxetine: Adjust dose in patients with impaired renal and hepatic function
Calcium-channel α-2-δ ligands • Gabapentin • Pregabalin	Acts on the α-2-δ subunit of voltage-gated calcium channels, decreasing central sensitization	Sedation, peripheral edema, weight gain, dizziness, incoordination	Gabapentin: 300–3600 mg divided 3 times daily Extended-release formulation available Pregabalin: 150–600 mg divided up to 3 times daily	Gabapentin: Adjust dose in patients with renal dysfunction Pregabalin: Adjust dose in patients with renal dysfunction Use with caution in patients with severe cardiovascular disease

(continued)

TABLE 8.5 Common Neuropathic Pain Medications (*continued*)

Drug	Mechanism of action	Side effects	Dosing range	Precautions
Opioid agonists • Tramadol • Tapentadol	μ-Receptor agonists; inhibit monoamine reuptake	Constipation, nausea and vomiting, dizziness, somnolence	Tramadol: 100–400 mg divided up to 4 times daily Tapentadol: 100–500 divided twice daily Extended-release formulation available	Tramadol: May lower seizure threshold Adjust dose in patients with renal dysfunction Tapentadol: Adjust dose in patients with hepatic dysfunction
Opioids (e.g., oxycodone, hydromorphone, morphine)	μ-Receptor agonists	Constipation, nausea, vomiting, dizziness, somnolence	Varies depending on formulation	
Alpha-lipoic acid	Antioxidant	Nausea, vomiting, dizziness, skin rash	600 mg daily in 2 divided doses	
Topical lidocaine patches	Sodium-channel blocker	Skin reactions including erythema/pruritus	Up to 3 patches on for 12 hours, off for 12 hours Also available as an ointment, cream, and gel	None
Capsaicin patches	Transient receptor potential vanilloid 1 (TRPV1) agonist	Associated allodynia initially, erythema, elevated blood pressure	Apply to affected area not more than 4 patches per application for 60 minutes Also available as an ointment that can be applied 4 times daily	Use with caution in patients with hypertension

the alpha-2-delta subunit of voltage-dependent calcium channels. Gabapentin is effective for painful diabetic neuropathy and postherpetic neuralgia, but appears to be less beneficial in chemotherapy-induced neuropathy and HIV neuropathy. It is considered a first-line treatment option in most conditions with neuropathic pain. The typical effective dose is between 1,800 and 3,600 mg/day, and it takes several weeks to titrate up the dose. Sedation is the most common side effect and can be mitigated by starting with a low dose and titrating slowly. Dizziness, weight gain, and edema may also occur. Pregabalin is like gabapentin and is approved by the FDA for the treatment of painful diabetic neuropathy and postherpetic neuralgia. Doses greater than 300 mg/day have not demonstrated significant additional benefit. Sedation, edema, dizziness, and weight gain are also side effects.

- Lidocaine 5% patches can alleviate pain in the location to which they are applied. They work by reducing ectopic discharges by blocking sodium channels. These patches are safe and well-tolerated given the minimal systemic absorption of lidocaine. Patches may be worn for 12 hours at a time and then should be removed for 12 hours.
- Capsaicin activates transient receptor potential vanilloid 1 (TRPV1) ligand-gated channels on nociceptive fibers. Depolarization follows, with transmission of pain signals to the spinal cord. The TRPV1 sensory axons become desensitized after several days, resulting in an inhibition of pain transmission. Capsaicin is available as an ointment and as patches. Some patients may choose not to continue with the therapy, as the cream causes severe burning during the first several days of application. The cream may require administration several times per day. A high-concentration patch (8%) may be worn for 30 to 60 minutes, resulting in benefits for several weeks. Capsaicin ointment and patches may cause erythema, edema, and pruritus. Patients may experience elevated blood pressure due to the severe pain in the first several days.
- Tramadol is a weak opioid μ-receptor agonist that also inhibits serotonin and norepinephrine reuptake. Tramadol's primary side effects include nausea, constipation, somnolence, dry mouth, and dizziness. Combination of tramadol with other serotonergic drugs should be avoided, as it may result in serotonin syndrome. Effective doses are usually 200 to 400 mg/day.

Disease-Specific Management

- Patients with poorly controlled type 1 diabetes mellitus are at higher risk of developing a neuropathy. Intensive glycemic control has been shown to delay the neuropathy onset in large observational studies. Pancreatic transplant and islet-cell transplantation may result in improvement of diabetic neuropathy—an outcome supported by improvement on neurophysiological studies. The data in type 2 diabetes are not as convincing, with several studies having demonstrated that intensive glycemic control is not associated with improvement in neuropathy. Diet and exercise, however, may delay the onset of neuropathy in patients with glucose intolerance and type 2 diabetes mellitus. In some studies, even though weight, glycemic control, and lipid parameters improved, neuropathy still developed and progressed.

- Once a vitamin deficiency is identified, supplementation is necessary. As the pathology in vitamin B_{12} deficiency is localized to the spinal cord and peripheral nerves, supplementation may halt progression of the disease, but may not reverse it. Similarly, in copper deficiency, the copper must be supplemented, and the cause of the copper deficiency (such as zinc toxicity resulting from excess use of denture cream) identified and addressed. As copper deficiency causes a myeloneuropathy, supplementation may arrest the progression, but not improve the disease. See Table 8.2 for recommended dosages for vitamin deficiency supplementation.

- The neuropathies discussed in this chapter that would be amenable to treatment with immunomodulatory or immunosuppressant medications include all neuropathies in the paraneoplastic category, neuropathies associated with primary rheumatologic diseases (e.g., Sjögren-associated sensory neuronopathy), sarcoidosis-associated neuropathies, the sensory form of CIDP, and CISP. Given the rarity of these diseases, there are no randomized-controlled treatment trials to guide management in these patients. Treatments that have been tried for these diseases include IVIG, plasma exchange, rituximab, corticosteroids, cyclophosphamide, mycophenolate mofetil, and azathioprine among others. One protocol for Sjögren-associated sensory neuronopathy recommends treating patients with IVIG (2 g/kg divided over 5 days, followed by monthly infusions). In patients with neurosarcoidosis and refractory disease, infliximab can also be considered. Refer to Table 8.6 for a discussion of commonly used immunotherapies.

- Treatment of infectious neuropathies is aimed at treating the infection itself. A discussion of antiviral therapies is beyond the scope of this chapter. Similarly, toxic neuropathies are treated by discontinuing the offending agent. Depending on the toxin, the neuropathy may improve, arrest, or even progress after withdrawal. The "coasting effect" in chemotherapy-induced neuropathies describes worsening of the neuropathy for several months following termination of the chemotherapeutic agent.

- The treatment of paraneoplastic neuropathies includes tumor treatment, immunomodulatory treatment, and symptomatic management. Tumor treatment may stabilize or even improve the

TABLE 8.6 Immunosuppressant Medications

Drug	Mechanism of action	Dose range	Side effects	Monitoring
Corticosteroids • Prednisone • Prednisolone • Methylprednisolone	• Decrease number of lymphocytes • Limit release of pro-inflammatory cytokines • Inhibit macrophage function • Reduce transmigration of lymphocytes	For prednisone and prednisolone, up to 1 mg/kg/day For refractory disease, consider IV methylprednisolone 1000 mg/day for 3–5 days. Weekly IV methylprednisolone may have a better side-effect profile for maintenance therapy.	Insomnia, GERD, Cushingoid features, osteopenia, weight gain, hyperglycemia, hypertension, thin skin, easy bruising, impaired would healing, gastritis, ulcer formation, cataracts, glaucoma, psychiatric disturbance, myopathy	• Height, weight, BMI, blood pressure • Glucose (hemoglobin A1c, fasting plasma glucose, oral glucose tolerance test) • Lipids • Annual bone density scan • Annual eye exam
Rituximab	• Chimeric anti-CD20 monoclonal immunoglobulin • Mediates complement-dependent cell lysis and antibody-dependent cytotoxicity	2 dosing regimens used • 375 mg/m² weekly × 4 weeks • 1 gram every other week × 2 doses • May repeat every 6–18 months for maintenance	Hypotension, nausea, vomiting, fever, dyspnea, angioedema, headache, urticaria, pulmonary disease, infections including progressive multifocal leukoencephalopathy	• PPD, hepatitis B and C testing prior to initiation • Flow cytometry for CD19, CD20 counts

(continued)

TABLE 8.6 Immunosuppressant Medications (*continued*)

Drug	Mechanism of action	Dose range	Side effects	Monitoring
Azathioprine	• Purine antimetabolite that inhibits B- and T-cell function	Goal dose range 2–3 mg/kg/day	Acute hypersensitivity reaction, liver toxicity, pancreatitis, bone marrow suppression, increased risk of infection, lymphoma, skin cancers, pancreatitis	CBC and liver enzymes weekly for the first month, then monthly for 6 months, then every 3 months
Methotrexate	• Folate-inhibiting drug	Start at 7.5–15 mg/week and gradually titrate up to 20–25 mg/week	Mucocutaneous problems, liver toxicity, gastrointestinal toxicity, bone marrow suppression, rash, increased risk of infection, interstitial pneumonitis	Liver function tests and CBC monitored closely
Mycophenolate mofetil	• Blocks B- and T-cell proliferation by inhibiting de novo pathway of purine nucleotide synthesis	Up to 2–3 g divided twice daily	Nausea, vomiting, diarrhea, headache, leukopenia, increased susceptibility to infection, tremor	CBC with differential monthly for 6 months, then every 3 months after
Cyclophosphamide	• Alkylating agent that targets proliferating B and T cells	1 g/m^2 IV monthly or 200 mg/kg IV divided over 4 days	Headache, nausea, rash, leukopenia, infertility, bone marrow suppression, hemorrhagic cystitis, malignancy	CBC with differential and urinalysis

(*continued*)

TABLE 8.6 Immunosuppressant Medications (*continued*)

Drug	Mechanism of action	Dose range	Side effects	Monitoring
Intravenous immune globulins (IVIG)	• Fc receptor blockade • Modulation of Fcγ receptor expression • Modulation of inflammatory response • Binding of anti-idiotypic antibodies to autoantibodies • Neutralization of complement factors • Targets B cell–activating factor	2 g/kg divided over 2–5 days; frequency and dosing of subsequent maintenance treatment individualized depending on response and relapses	Anaphylaxis in IgA deficiency, aseptic meningitis, headache, flu-like reaction, rash, neutropenia, hyperviscosity syndrome, renal insufficiency, fluid overload	May check an IgA level before initiation
Plasma exchange	• Removal of pathogenic antibodies form the blood	One plasma volume per exchange procedure for 3–5 days	Line-related infections, bleeding, thrombosis, hypotension, hypocalcemia, hemolysis, anemia	Coagulation studies during periods of exchange

BMI, body mass index; CBC, complete blood count; GERD, gastroesophageal reflux disease; IgA, immunoglobulin A; PPD, purified protein derivative.

paraneoplastic disease. The different immunomodulatory thera-pies described earlier have been tried with varying degrees of suc-cess. Patients with early disease and mild disability may experience more improvement. A guideline has been published that recom-mends anti-Hu and anti-CRMP-5/CV2 paraneoplastic syndromes be treated with high-dose corticosteroids and/or IVIG, followed by cyclophosphamide in the absence of identifiable malignancy. The prognosis for patients with paraneoplastic sensory neuronopathy is quite poor, with the median survival being less than 1 year.

- Treatment of AL amyloid includes chemotherapeutic agents aimed at eliminating the plasma cell clone and stem cell trans-plantation. High-dose melphalan and subsequent autologous stem cell transplant have been shown to be effective. Patients will demonstrate improvement in their sensory and autonomic neuropathy. Additional chemotherapeutic therapies being investi-gated for AL amyloidosis include bortezomib, cyclophosphamide, and dexamethasone.

- The mainstay of treatment in transthyretin familial amyloidosis has been orthotopic liver transplant. This procedure removes the mutant transthyretin and prevents further accumulation of amy-loid deposits. The Val30Met genotype tends to benefit greatest from liver transplant. Both the neuropathy and the cardiomyop-athy may continue to worsen following liver transplantation. Taf-amidis, which is a transthyretin stabilizer, is available in Europe, but is not yet FDA approved. It has been demonstrated to slow the rate of neurologic progression and is most efficacious if started early in the disease.

- Fabry disease is a treatable lysosomal storage disorder. The two treatments are recombinant human alpha-Gal A enzyme replace-ment therapies (agalsidase beta and agalsidase alfa), but only agalsidase beta is FDA approved for use in the United States. These enzyme replacement therapies have reported benefit in control of neuropathic pain.

- The treatment of postherpetic neuralgia has been well studied and focuses on symptom management. For mild pain, topical treatment with lidocaine patches, capsaicin cream, and especially the higher-concentration formulation (8%) capsaicin patches is appropriate. Appropriate systemic treatments for postherpetic neuralgia pain include tricyclic antidepressants, gabapentin, and the FDA-approved pregabalin. Opioids and tramadol should be considered third-line therapies. In terms of prevention, the live attenuated VZV vaccine is available to all patients 50 years and older. In those who have received the vaccine, the incidence of postherpetic neuralgia decreases by nearly 70%.

- Treatment of trigeminal neuralgia includes the antiepileptic drugs, classically carbamazepine. Nearly one-third of patients will initially be resistant to carbamazepine; in such cases, alternative medications such as baclofen, oxcarbazepine, gabapentin, topiramate, and lamotrigine may be used. Botulinum toxin injections may be beneficial in trigeminal neuralgia. For those patients who are medically refractory, surgical therapy in the form of microvascular decompression and ganglion-level ablative procedures are options.

- Treatment of autoimmune trigeminal neuropathy has included corticosteroids, which have led to a little improvement in a few reported cases. When a structural lesion is identified compressing the trigeminal nerve, surgical intervention might be necessary.

CONCLUSION

The presentations of sensory-predominant nerve diseases are diverse and dictated largely by which component of the sensory nervous system is involved. Most of these sensory neuropathies are part of a spectrum, affecting combinations of fiber types (e.g., small fiber and autonomic, sensorimotor, DRG, and autonomic). Even so, understanding the patient's primary complaint—that is, "burning pain" or "gait imbalance"—and pertinent examination findings will guide the physician to a category of diseases based on localization, and will dictate appropriate diagnostic workup and treatment.

SUGGESTED READING

Cortez M, Singleton JR, Smith AG. Glucose intolerance, metabolic syndrome, and neuropathy. *Handb Clin Neurol.* 2014;126:109–122.

Finnerup NB, Attal N, Haroutounian S, et al. Pharmacotherapy for neuropathic pain in adults: a systemic review and meta-analysis. *Lancet Neurol.* 2015;14(2):162–173.

Gibbons CH, Freeman R. Treatment-induced neuropathy of diabetes: an acute, iatrogenic complication of diabetes. *Brain.* 2015;138(Pt 1): 43–52.

Gwathmey KG. Sensory neuronopathies. *Muscle Nerve.* 2016;53(1): 8–19.

Johnson RW, Rice AS. Clinical practice: postherpetic neuralgia. *N Engl J Med.* 2014;371(16):1526–1533.

Oaklander AL. Immunotherapy prospects for painful small-fiber sensory neuropathies and ganglionopathies. *Neurotherapeutics.* 2016;13(1):108–117.

Reddy GD, Viswanathan A. Trigeminal and glossopharyngeal neuralgia. *Neurol Clin.* 2014;32(2):539–552.

Smith JH, Cutrer FM. Numbness matters: a clinical review of trigeminal neuropathy. *Cephalalgia.* 2011;31(10):1131–1144.

Yuki N, Uncini A. Acute and chronic ataxic neuropathies with disialosyl antibodies: a continuous clinical spectrum and a common pathophysiological mechanism. *Muscle Nerve.* 2014;49(5):629–635.

9 Limb Pain

Andrew W. Tarulli

HISTORY

- Limb pain is a common complaint evaluated by neurologists. Knowledge of both neurologic and musculoskeletal sources of limb pain is necessary to make the correct diagnosis and determine an appropriate treatment plan.
- Traumatic injuries to the limbs are common, but generally not managed by neurologists. Unless there is specific damage to a component of the nervous system, traumatic injuries are not discussed in detail in this chapter.
- The initial step in determining the origin of limb pain is to define the distribution of symptoms.
  - Arm pain can be divided into shoulder-girdle pain, humeral pain, elbow pain, forearm pain, hand pain, and finger pain.
  - Leg pain can be divided into hip pain, thigh pain, knee pain, lower leg pain, foot pain, and toe pain.
- The next step is to define the quality and tempo of the pain.
- Pain secondary to damage to the nerve, including the nerve roots, nerve plexi, and peripheral nerves themselves, is usually characterized by sharp, burning, or electrical qualities. It tends to be worse with rest or when ambient stimuli are removed (e.g., when trying to fall asleep). Pressure on a nerve may aggravate pain if the site of nerve injury is close to the skin surface.
  - Ischemia of the nerve classically produces pain that is sudden in onset, and is often associated with dense weakness in that nerve's motor distribution.
  - Inflammation of the nerve may produce either sudden-onset or gradual-onset pain.
  - Compression of the nerve typically produces pain that develops slowly and progresses over time.

- Pain secondary to musculoskeletal disorders is usually character-ized by tight, sore, or aching qualities. The pain is aggravated by use or overuse of the affected region and often improves with rest.
- Pain secondary to vascular disorders is often accompanied by a sense of coldness in the extremity, tingling, mottling of the skin, or weakness of peripheral pulses.

CLINICAL INVESTIGATION

- After the history is obtained, clinical investigation begins with care-ful neuromuscular, musculoskeletal, and vascular examination.
- The location of the pain (described in the previous section) guides clinical investigation.
- In patients with suspected peripheral nervous system disorders, electromyography (EMG) and nerve conduction studies (NCS) may be helpful in diagnosis. Electrodiagnostic testing must always be informed by the history and neurologic examination: "Fishing trips" are not likely to lead to a diagnosis. When arrang-ing for EMG and NCS to investigate a peripheral nerve disorder, it is important to allow ample time for the lesion to reach electro-physiologic maturity, which usually occurs at 3 weeks after onset.
  - NCS may identify a site of a peripheral nerve lesion by demon-strating slowed conduction velocity or conduction block across a compression site or region of inflamed nerve.
  - The earliest needle EMG sign of nerve injury is reduced motor unit recruitment, which occurs immediately after nerve injury. Between 1 and 3 weeks following a nerve injury, EMG may show denervation in the form of fibrillation potentials and pos-itive sharp waves. After 3 months, EMG may show chronic rein-nervation in the form of large amplitude, long duration, and polyphasic motor units.
- Imaging studies are useful for specific neurologic injuries involv-ing the limbs:
  - Magnetic resonance imaging (MRI) of the cervical or lumbosa-cral spine can identify nerve root pathologies. Because these are mostly compressive in nature, contrast enhancement is typically not required. Infectious and neoplastic radiculopa-thies, however, may require the addition of contrast.
  - MRI of the shoulder or pelvis can identify compression, infil-tration, or inflammation of the brachial or lumbosacral plexus. Contrast administration is usually required.
  - Computed tomography (CT) scan of the pelvis is often useful for patients with lumbosacral plexopathy due to retroperito-neal hematoma.
  - Nerve ultrasound is being employed with increasing frequency and is capable of identifying nerve injuries at sites that are

usually not well visualized with other imaging modalities or electrophysiologic techniques.

- Imaging studies of the appropriate joint or region of soft-tissue injury can be helpful for patients with musculoskeletal disorders. Typically, imaging starts with plain x-rays to evaluate for bony trauma and degenerative changes; if these are not revealing, the clinician should proceed to MRI to evaluate the soft tissues in greater detail.
- Evaluation of vascular injuries is usually conducted by a specialist in vascular medicine or surgery. Studies including arteriograms, venograms, Doppler ultrasounds, and ankle-brachial indices are helpful in pinpointing sites of vascular blockage.

DIFFERENTIAL DIAGNOSIS
Upper Extremity
Because they can produce pain in any part of the upper limb, cervical radiculopathies and brachial plexopathies will be discussed first, before moving on to a discussion of conditions that affect specific parts of the upper limb.

Cervical Radiculopathies
- Cervical radiculopathies typically produce pain and paresthesias in a radiating fashion—for example, from the neck into the arm. Alternatively, the pain may radiate upward from the arm into the neck or the neck may be completely uninvolved.
- Table 9.1 provides a summary of the dermatomes of the upper extremity. Symptoms frequently do not conform to these dermatomes. For example, a patient with a C5 radiculopathy may have pain throughout the arm rather than in just the classical C5 distribution of the superolateral shoulder.
- Table 9.2 provides a summary of the myotomes of the upper extremity. The muscles listed represent a small, clinically useful sample of muscles that can be examined quickly at the bedside.
- The most common source of upper-extremity radiculopathies is degenerative disease of the cervical spine: A herniated nucleus pulposus compresses the traversing or exiting nerve root and

TABLE 9.1 Dermatomes of the Upper Extremity

Dermatome	Cutaneous innervation
C5	Lateral shoulder and upper arm
C6	Lateral forearm, digits 1 and 2
C7	Digit 3
C8	Medial forearm, digits 4 and 5
T1	Medial upper arm

TABLE 9.2 Myotomes of the Upper Extremity	
Myotome	**Muscular innervation**
C5	Deltoid, biceps
C6	Deltoid, biceps, triceps, flexor carpi radialis
C7	Triceps, flexor carpi radialis, extensor carpi radialis, extensor digitorum communis
C8	Abductor digiti minimi, abductor pollicis brevis, first dorsal interosseous
T1	Abductor digiti minimi, abductor pollicis brevis, first dorsal interosseous

results in arm pain and other radicular symptoms. Spinal stenosis with bony and ligamentous hypertrophy may also compress the nerve root, and is more common in older patients.

▪ For most patients with degenerative disease, conservative therapy including a soft cervical collar, a brief course of nonsteroidal anti-inflammatory drugs (NSAIDs), and light physical therapy will be effective. Epidural steroid injections may be helpful for patients whose condition fails to resolve with conservative measures. Surgery is reserved for patients with refractory pain, progressive weakness, or coexisting myelopathy.

● Infection of the nerve root without degenerative disc disease may also produce radiculopathies. Common infections of the nerve root include:

▪ Neuroborreliosis (Lyme disease). Lyme disease is a multisystem tick-borne infection caused by *Borrelia burgdorferi*. Radiculo-neuritis is an uncommon but classical neurologic manifestation. It is diagnosed by finding elevated immunoglobulin M (IgM) antibodies to *B. burgdorferi* in the serum or cerebrospinal fluid. In approximately 50% of cases, though, radiculitis is an early manifestation of *Borrelia* infection, and antibody results will be negative. Treatment options include intravenous ceftriaxone 2 g daily × 14 to 21 days or doxycycline 200 to 400 mg daily × 21 to 42 days.

▪ Herpes zoster (shingles). Reactivation of latent varicella zoster virus in the dorsal root ganglia produces herpes zoster, also known as shingles. This disease is characterized by a painful, blistering rash that affects the distribution of a single nerve root or sometimes several adjacent nerve roots. Immunocompetent patients may develop pain without a rash, so-called zoster sine herpete. Treatment options include acyclovir 800 mg five times per day × 7 days, famciclovir 500 mg three times per day × 7 days, or valacyclovir 1,000 mg three times per day × 7 days.

- Both primary and metastatic tumors may affect the nerve roots.
  - Primary tumors that affect the nerve roots include schwannoma, neurofibroma, meningioma, and ependymoma.
  - Metastases to nerve roots typically affect the adjacent spinal cord as well, potentially leading to cord compression that overshadows the radiculopathic component of the presentation.

Brachial Plexopathy

- Trauma, compression, inflammation, or infiltration of the brachial plexus may produce arm pain. The entire brachial plexus may be involved, or the lesion may be patchy and involve only a portion of the plexus, such as the upper or lower trunk.
- Electrophysiologic evaluation can be very helpful in distinguishing a brachial plexopathy from a cervical radiculopathy.
  - In both brachial plexopathy and cervical radiculopathy, motor NCS will be abnormal, demonstrating reduced compound muscle action potentials.
  - Because the pathology in a brachial plexopathy is distal to the dorsal root ganglion, sensory NCS will be abnormal in a brachial plexopathy. In most cervical radiculopathies (including essentially all radiculopathies due to structural disease), the pathology occurs proximal to the dorsal root ganglion, leading to normal sensory NCS.
  - It may be difficult to distinguish brachial plexopathy from cervical radiculopathy using EMG, as denervation and reinnervation in the distribution of multiple nerve roots and individual nerves will be identified in either condition.
- Idiopathic brachial neuritis (i.e., brachial plexitis or Parsonage-Turner syndrome) is characterized by the acute or subacute onset of pain and paresthesias in the arm, followed days to weeks later by muscle weakness. It is seen most often as an autoimmune response to a viral infection or immunization. There is a predilection for involvement of the suprascapular nerve, the long thoracic nerve, and the anterior interosseous nerve. In most cases, imaging studies, including dedicated MRI of the brachial plexus with and without contrast, are normal. Unfortunately, no treatment has proved effective in reversing the symptoms of idiopathic brachial neuritis, and time to allow nerve repair is the only effective treatment.
- Malignant infiltration is another possible etiology of brachial plexopathy. Tumors, especially lung and breast tumors, can metastasize to the brachial plexus. Classically, the infiltration involves the lower trunk or the entire plexus and results in severe pain that interferes with sleep. The pain can involve the entire arm or just a single region within the arm. After several weeks, progressive muscle weakness

and atrophy develops. Brachial plexopathy due to malignant infiltration is a poor prognostic sign, and treatment should focus on pain control. Palliative radiation is often used to achieve this.

- Radiation-induced plexopathy is also possible. Radiation used to treat thoracic or mediastinal tumors such as lung cancer, breast cancer, and lymphoma may result in brachial plexopathy. The pain is typically mild and less prominent than the pain of plexopathy due to malignant infiltration. Myokymia, a twitching or wriggling of muscles underneath the skin, may be identified clinically or electromyographically, and is an important sign of a radiation-induced plexopathy. Unfortunately, treatment options for radiation-induced plexopathy are limited.

Shoulder

Rotator Cuff Tendinopathy and Subacromial Bursitis

- The muscles and tendons of the rotator cuff of the shoulder are the supraspinatus, infraspinatus, teres minor, and subscapularis. Overuse of the shoulder can result in rotator cuff tendonitis or tear. Inflammation of the subacromial bursa, which overlies the supraspinatus, may produce similar symptoms. Pain is localized to the shoulder and upper arm. Patients often complain of shoulder weakness, which is actually due to instability at the site of the tendon.
- On physical examination, several maneuvers may provoke the pain of rotator cuff tendonitis or subacromial bursitis, thereby confirming the diagnosis.
  - Hawkins' test is positive when internal rotation of the humerus elicits pain while the shoulder and elbow are flexed.
  - The empty can test is positive when pronation of the forearm and internal rotation of the humerus elicits pain while the shoulder is abducted and the elbow is extended.
  - Neer's test is positive when forward flexion at the shoulder produces pain when the arm is internally rotated.
- MRI can be useful to confirm the diagnosis when the results of the physical examination are unclear or if surgery is being contemplated.
- Physical therapy, NSAIDs, and local steroid injections may help relieve pain. If these therapies are not effective, then surgery can be considered.

Forearm

Lateral Epicondylitis

- Inflammation of the extensor carpi radialis tendons at their insertion on the humerus leads to lateral epicondylitis (tennis elbow). Patients complain of pain in the lateral forearm and elbow, which occurs with overuse.

- The pain may be elicited by palpation of the extensor tendons in the proximal lateral forearm, by forced wrist extension, or by attempting to lift a chair with the wrist pronated.
- Treatment consists of rest, stretching exercises, and local massage. Surgery is rarely required.

Medial Epicondylitis

- Inflammation of the flexor carpi radialis tendon at its insertion on the humerus leads to medial epicondylitis (golfer's elbow). Patients complain of pain localized to the medial forearm.
- The pain may be reproduced by palpation of the flexor tendons at the proximal medial forearm, by forced wrist flexion, or by attempting to lift a chair with the arm supinated.
- Treatment consists of rest, stretching exercises, and local massage. Surgery is rarely required.

Posterior Interosseous Neuropathy

- The posterior interosseous nerve is the principal motor branch of the radial nerve. It divides from the radial nerve proper in the distal upper arm and innervates the extensor muscles of the wrist and fingers, the supinator, and the abductor pollicis longus. It does not have a sensory branch.
- There are two classical entrapment sites of the posterior interosseous nerve:
  - The radial tunnel in the lateral intermuscular septum of the arm between the brachialis and brachioradialis muscles (radial tunnel syndrome)
  - The arcade of Frohse in the superficial head of the supinator muscle (supinator syndrome)
- Both the radial tunnel and supinator syndromes are rare and controversial diagnoses. In both cases, pain is dull and aching, involves the proximal dorsal forearm, and is aggravated by movement. Weakness may be due to pain limitation or due to involvement of the motor branches of the nerve. There is no sensory loss because the posterior interosseous nerve is a pure motor nerve.
- Nerve blockade or decompression of the posterior interosseous nerve at the supinator may lead to clinical improvement.

Hand

Neurogenic Thoracic Outlet Syndrome

- This rare disorder is caused by compression of the lower trunk of the brachial plexus, most often by an accessory rib but sometimes by a hypertrophied scalene muscle or band of connective tissue. The potential for repetitive injury to cause the syndrome without anatomic compression is controversial. This syndrome is overdiagnosed: Many patients with upper extremity pain of unclear etiology are misdiagnosed with thoracic outlet syndrome.

- Typical symptoms are pain and numbness in the medial hand and forearm. Weakness of intrinsic muscles of the hand accompanies the pain.
- The subclavian artery and vein may also be compromised, resulting in a vascular or combined neurovascular thoracic outlet syndrome. When severe, there may be pulselessness and bluish discoloration in the affected arm when it is raised overhead.
- The electrophysiologic findings of neurogenic thoracic outlet syndrome are reduced compound motor action potentials (CMAPs) in the median and ulnar nerve and reduced sensory nerve action potentials (SNAPs) in the ulnar nerve. The median SNAP is normal because this portion of the nerve is not derived from the lower trunk of the brachial plexus.
- Treatment includes physical therapy and pain relief with NSAIDs. Surgical decompression is employed for patients with refractory pain.

Carpometacarpal Arthritis

- Osteoarthritis of the first carpometacarpal joint is very common in older patients.
- Pain at the base of the thumb may occur on both the palmar and dorsal aspects of the hand. On examination, compression of the carpometacarpal joint in the anterior–posterior direction reproduces the pain.
- Carpometacarpal arthritis should be treated with rest, NSAIDs, and a thumb spica splint for immobilization.

De Quervain Tenosynovitis

- Inflammation of the distal tendons of the abductor pollicis longus and extensor pollicis produces de Quervain tenosynovitis.
- Pain is located at the base of the thumb and radiates into the distal radial forearm. The Finkelstein maneuver, in which pain is reproduced by enclosing the thumb in the fist and deviating it in the ulnar direction, is diagnostic.
- Patients respond to immobilization with a thumb spica splint and NSAIDs.

Flexor Tenosynovitis (Trigger Finger)

- Inflammation of the flexor tendons of the fingers may produce pain in the palmar surface of the hand, though locking of the fingers in flexion is often more prominent.
- On examination, symptoms can be reproduced by applying pressure to the palm superficial to the involved tendon.

- Occupational therapy and NSAIDs can be helpful, but local steroid injections or surgical release are often necessary.

Carpal Tunnel Syndrome

- Carpal tunnel syndrome (CTS) is the set of clinical findings caused by compression of the median nerve at the wrist. Typically, the compression occurs as part of a wear-and-tear degenerative process. Risk factors for carpal tunnel syndrome include excessive manual work (especially with vibrating machinery), hypothyroidism, rheumatoid arthritis, amyloidosis, and pregnancy.
- The most common symptoms of CTS are tingling and numbness in the thumb, index finger, middle finger, and lateral half of the ring finger. Some patients describe these paresthesias as painful. Although the palmar surface of the fingers should be involved and the dorsum of the hand should be spared, many patients describe symptoms in the entire palm, dorsum of the hand, and even the forearm. Symptoms tend to be worse at night or with overuse.
- On examination, weakness of thumb abduction may be identified. Muscles derived from the median nerve proximal to the carpal tunnel (e.g., flexor carpi radialis) and anterior interosseous branch of the median nerve (e.g., flexor pollicis longus) are spared. Sensory loss involves the palmar aspects of digits 1 to 3 and the median half of digit 4. The Tinel sign is positive when tapping the volar surface of the wrist elicits paresthesias in digits 1 to 4. The Phalen sign is positive when the patient develops paresthesias in this distribution when the dorsal surfaces of both hands are opposed. The flick sign is positive when the patient shakes out the hand to relieve the paresthesias.
- Carpal tunnel syndrome can be confirmed electrodiagnostically.
  - The cornerstone of the electrodiagnosis of CTS is finding evidence for slowing of median nerve conduction velocity across the wrist. This can be identified using routine sensory and motor NCS. In more subtle cases, comparison studies are required: Relative slowing of median nerve conduction velocity compared to ulnar or radial nerve (which supply sensorimotor function to the hand but do not traverse the carpal tunnel) conduction velocity will be identified.
  - Needle EMG may show denervation or reinnervation of median-innervated muscles distal to the carpal tunnel, most commonly the abductor pollicis brevis, with sparing of muscles that have more proximal origins from the median nerve, such as the flexor carpi radialis.
- Treatment of carpal tunnel syndrome begins by avoiding provoking or exacerbating activities. If this is not possible or successful, then splinting of the hands, particularly at night, may be helpful. Injection of corticosteroids in the carpal tunnel may help to

relieve inflammation. For patients with refractory carpal tunnel syndrome, surgical decompression is quite effective.

Ulnar Neuropathy at the Elbow

- Compression of the ulnar nerve at the elbow, usually by a gradual wear-and-tear process, can lead to pain, numbness, and tingling in the medial hand and digits 4 and 5.
- On examination, weakness of intrinsic hand muscles innervated by the ulnar nerve, including the abductor digiti minimi and the first dorsal interosseous, supports the diagnosis of ulnar neuropathy at the elbow. In severe cases, these muscles will atrophy. Muscles with more proximal innervation from the ulnar nerve, including the flexor carpi ulnaris and flexor digitorum profundus 4 + 5, may also be involved. A reduction in sensation over the fifth digit and medial fourth digit and the adjacent palm suggests the diagnosis. Because the dorsal ulnar cutaneous nerve branches off distal to the elbow, sensation will be impaired on both the dorsal and palmar aspects of the hand. The ulnar Tinel sign is positive when percussion of the nerve at the elbow produces paresthesias in digits 4 and 5.
- Ulnar neuropathy at the elbow can be confirmed electrophysiologically by finding evidence for slowing of motor conduction velocity across the elbow. Needle EMG may show denervation or reinnervation of all ulnar-innervated muscles (there are no muscles innervated by the ulnar nerve that arise proximal to the elbow).
- Treatment of ulnar neuropathy at the elbow begins with wearing a protective elbow sleeve during activities that aggravate the neuropathy and at night. If this is unsuccessful, surgical decompression or transposition of the nerve should be pursued.

Ulnar Neuropathy at the Wrist

- Compression of the ulnar nerve at the wrist (Guyon's canal) is much less common than compression at the elbow. Branches of the ulnar nerve that are proximal to the wrist (motor branches to the flexors of the fourth and fifth digits and flexors of the forearm, and the dorsal ulnar cutaneous nerve) are spared.
- Risk factors for ulnar neuropathy at the wrist include bicycle riding and using a walker. A ganglion cyst of the nerve may also produce an ulnar neuropathy at the wrist.
- An ulnar nerve lesion at Guyon's canal may occur at one of the three sites.
    - Type I lesions occur proximally in Guyon's canal and affect both the superficial and deep branches of the ulnar nerve. All motor ulnar nerve function and sensation to the hypothenar eminence and digits 4 and 5 are affected.

- Type II lesions occur within Guyon's canal and affect only the deep branch of the nerve, leading to motor dysfunction only. Sensation is preserved.
- Type III lesions occur in the distal portion of Guyon's canal and affect only sensation to the hypothenar eminence and digits 4 and 5.
- Electrophysiologic confirmation of an ulnar neuropathy at Guyon's canal involves finding prolonged ulnar latencies compared to median latencies across the wrist. This is most commonly done by comparing the onset latencies of the ulnar-innervated first palmar interosseous to the median-innervated second lumbrical.
- Ulnar neuropathy at the wrist can be treated by avoiding provocative activities. If applicable, ganglion cyst drainage or removal should be performed.

Lower Extremity
Radiculopathies of the Lower Extremity

- Compression or inflammation of the lumbosacral nerve roots is a very common source of lower back and leg pain.
- The structural and inflammatory diseases that affect the lumbosacral nerve roots are similar to those that affect the cervical nerve roots. See the earlier section on cervical radiculopathies for general comments on radiculopathies that also apply to lumbosacral radiculopathies.
- Table 9.3 provides a summary of the dermatomes of the lower extremity.
- Table 9.4 provides a summary of the myotomes of the lower extremity.
- In addition to sensorimotor dysfunction of the nerves and muscles in the legs, pathology of the lumbosacral nerve roots may produce a cauda equina syndrome, in which sphincter function and perineal sensation are affected. Cauda equina syndrome is a surgical emergency when it is caused by structural compression such as by a herniated disc, osteoarthritis, hematoma, or a tumor.

TABLE 9.3 Dermatomes of the Lower Extremity

Dermatome	Cutaneous innervation
L2	Lateral thigh
L3	Medial thigh
L4	Medial lower leg
L5	Lateral lower leg, dorsal foot
S1	Lateral foot, calf

TABLE 9.4 Myotomes of the Lower Extremity	
Myotome	Muscular innervation
L2	Iliopsoas, quadriceps, adductor longus
L3	Iliopsoas, quadriceps, adductor longus
L4	Quadriceps, tibialis anterior
L5	Tibialis anterior, tibialis posterior, extensor hallucis longus
S1	Gastrocnemius, hamstrings

- Uncommon but characteristic infectious processes of the lumbosacral nerve roots and cauda equina are cytomegalovirus in patients with HIV infection and herpes simplex virus 2 (Elsberg syndrome).

Lumbosacral Plexopathy

- Disorders of the lumbosacral plexus produce leg pain as one of the major symptoms. Pathologies that affect the brachial plexus, including trauma, inflammation, and neoplasms also affect the lumbosacral plexus. The following are important conditions specific to the lumbosacral plexus:

  ▪ Diabetic amyotrophy (diabetic lumbosacral radiculoplexus neuropathy). This inflammatory disorder affects the lumbosacral nerve roots, plexus, and nerves derived from the plexus. It is associated with type 2 diabetes, and may be the first symptom of diabetes. Systemic symptoms including fever and weight loss may precede or develop simultaneously with the neuropathic symptoms. Most commonly, pain involves the pelvic region or proximal leg at onset, although symptoms may also occur distally in the leg. The pain can be intense and keep the patient awake at night. After several weeks, weakness and then atrophy develop in the affected leg. Symptoms may spread to the contralateral leg. There is no proven treatment for diabetic amyotrophy, and it may result in long-term disability.

  ▪ Idiopathic lumbosacral plexopathy. This clinical syndrome is similar to diabetic amyotrophy but a history of diabetes is absent. As with diabetic amyotrophy, there is no proven treatment for idiopathic lumbosacral plexopathy.

  ▪ Retroperitoneal hematoma. Hemorrhage into the lumbosacral plexus—a phenomenon often in patients who are taking blood thinners—is another source of lumbosacral plexopathy. The diagnosis is usually confirmed with CT scan of the pelvis. Treatment includes discontinuation of blood thinners and sometimes surgical evacuation in patients with severe plexus compression.

▪ Neoplasm-associated lumbosacral plexopathy. Colon, prostate, bladder, and gynecologic malignancies are the tumors that most commonly infiltrate the lumbosacral plexus. See the earlier section on brachial plexopathies for more specific comments concerning plexopathies due to direct neoplastic infiltration and to radiation damage.

Hip

Osteoarthritis of the Hip

- In general, neurologists diagnose osteoarthritis of the hip only when it is confused with another condition such as lumbosacral radiculopathy or lumbosacral plexopathy. Osteoarthritis of the hip is extremely common in older patients and develops by a wear-and-tear degenerative process that occurs over the course of many years. Pain may be located in the hip or be most prominent in the groin or thigh. The pain is often accompanied by a reduced range of motion and sometimes by a perception of weakness in the hip.

- The presence of osteoarthritis can be confirmed by plain x-rays of the hip. Because osteoarthritis is so common in older patients, any abnormal imaging studies should be interpreted judiciously.

- Conservative therapy begins with acetaminophen and NSAIDs. Glucosamine and chondroitin are often prescribed, but their benefit in treating osteoarthritis is unclear. Referral to an orthopedic surgeon may be needed when pain is refractory to conservative measures.

Avascular Necrosis (Osteonecrosis) of the Hip

- Avascular necrosis is caused by a lack of blood supply leading to progressive destruction of the bones of the hip joint. Initial symptoms include pain in the hip, groin, and buttock. If it progresses, avascular necrosis may cause bone weakness to the point of fracture and collapse.

- Risk factors for avascular necrosis include prior trauma, excessive alcohol use, and steroid use. It is, therefore, an important condition to consider in patients with neurologic disease who require long-term steroid administration, such as patients with myasthenia gravis, chronic inflammatory demyelinating polyradiculoneuropathy, inflammatory myopathy, and multiple sclerosis.

- The diagnosis can be established by imaging studies including x-ray, MRI, or bone scan.

- Treatment starts with risk factor modification. Rest and physical therapy can be effective for patients with mild disease. Core decompression is a surgical procedure in which necrotic bone is removed, thereby allowing healthy bone to grow in its place.

Outcomes of this procedure are mixed. Joint replacement is necessary for patients with severe disease.

Trochanteric Bursitis

- The trochanteric bursa lies superficial to the greater trochanter and head of the femur and deep to the gluteal muscles. Chronic wear-and-tear or pressure on the lateral hip leads to inflammation of this bursa, known as trochanteric bursitis.
- The pain tends to be worse when the patient sleeps on the side. In many instances, the pain is severe to the degree that the patient cannot sleep on the side at all.
- The diagnosis is confirmed by demonstrating tenderness to palpation at the trochanteric bursa. Neuroimaging studies are not typically needed, but ultrasound and MRI can be useful in ambiguous cases.
- Lying on the back or the unaffected side can be helpful. Pain relievers, heat, and stretching are often helpful. Steroid injections in the trochanteric bursa may be required for patients with refractory disease.

Foot

Plantar Fasciitis

- Degeneration and inflammation of the plantar fascia in the sole of the foot is a common condition in runners, overweight people, and people who work on their feet.
- The pain is localized to the sole of the foot and typically has a stabbing or burning quality. Classically, the symptoms are worst when first placing weight on the foot in the morning. The pain often makes walking difficult.
- The diagnosis can be confirmed by finding point tenderness of the plantar fascia with direct palpation. Plain films of the feet are sometimes performed to exclude calcaneal spurs, which may produce very similar pain.
- NSAIDs, physical therapy, and foot orthotics can help to relieve the pain. For patients with refractory pain, steroid injections can be helpful, although these injections may cause further deterioration of the plantar fascia. Rarely, surgical decompression is indicated.

Morton's Neuroma

- Injury or irritation of the interdigital nerves at the heads of the metatarsal bones produces pain in the sole of the foot. Risk factors for Morton's neuroma include wearing high heels and excessive pressure applied to the sole of the foot. While the pain may be described as diffuse, it is typically localized to the interdigital space, most commonly between the third and fourth toes. The pain may be exquisite, and patients often ask to not have their feet palpated for fear that this action will provoke their pain.

- The diagnosis can be confirmed radiologically by ultrasound or MRI of the foot.
- Conservative treatment includes shoe inserts to provide arch support and shock absorption. Switching from high heels to flat shoes can be helpful. Local steroid injections around the involved nerve can be effective when conservative therapy fails. Surgical decompression is reserved for refractory cases.

Multifocal Limb Pain Syndromes
Fibromyalgia

- Fibromyalgia is a chronic pain syndrome characterized by multiple points of tenderness in the neck, middle back, lower back, chest wall, arms, and legs. Numbness, tingling, burning, and muscle aches are common. The condition is six times more common in women than in men. Associated symptoms include irritable bowel, pelvic pain, interstitial cystitis, fatigue, anxiety, depression, memory loss, and impaired concentration. Many patients have more than 20 different symptoms.
- The diagnosis is established by history and excluding other diagnostic mimics. In many cases, this leads to prolonged diagnostic workups that disclose minor abnormalities, purely by statistical error. Patients often cling to these abnormalities as the source of their problem.
- Treatment is often not successful. Education about the chronic, unknown, irreversible nature of the condition is important. Other mainstays of treatment include physical therapy, antidepressants, and medications for neuropathic pain such as duloxetine, gabapentin, pregabalin, and topiramate. The effectiveness of any of these treatments, however, is modest.

Myofascial Pain Syndrome

- Myofascial pain is characterized by unexplained pain restricted to a single muscle or muscle group. The pain is usually worsened by activity of that muscle group. Trigger points, in which pressure applied to the painful area produces paresthesias, are observed.
- Similar to fibromyalgia, myofascial pain syndrome is a diagnosis of exclusion.
- Treatment is similar to that described for fibromyalgia. Other treatments that may be effective include physical therapy with local application of heat and ultrasound, as well as trigger point injections.

SUGGESTED READING

Dyck PJ, Windebank AJ. Diabetic and nondiabetic lumbosacral radiculoplexus neuropathies: new insights into pathophysiology and treatment. *Muscle Nerve*. 2002;25(4):477–491.

Eberhardt O, Kuker W, Dichgans J, Weller M. HSV-2 sacral radiculitis (Elsberg syndrome). *Neurology*. 2004;63(4):758–759.

Griffin LY. *Essentials of Musculoskeletal Care*. 3rd ed. Rosemont, IL: American Academy of Orthopaedic Surgeons; 2005.

Halperin JJ. Nervous system disease. *Infect Dis Clin North Am*. 2015;29(2):241–253.

Jaeckle KA. Neurologic manifestations of neoplastic and radiation-induced plexopathies. *Semin Neurol*. 2010;30(3):254–262.

Lee MW, McPhee RW, Stringer MD. An evidence-based approach to human dermatomes. *Clin Anat*. 2008;21(5):363–373.

Polston DW. Cervical radiculopathy. *Neurol Clin*. 2007;25(2):373–385.

Tarulli AW, Raynor EM. Lumbosacral radiculopathy. *Neurol Clin*. 2007;25(2):387–405.

Tsao BE, Ferrante MA, Wilbourn AJ, Shields RW. Electrodiagnostic features of true neurogenic thoracic outlet syndrome. *Muscle Nerve*. 2014;49(5):724–727.

White KP, Nielson WR, Harth M, et al. Does the label "fibromyalgia" alter health status, function, and health service utilization? A prospective, within-group comparison in a community cohort of adults with chronic widespread pain. *Arthritis Rheum*. 2002;47(3):260–265.

Index

weakness. *See also* acute
generalized weakness;
bulbar weakness; chronically
developing weakness;
episodic weakness; ocular
weakness; subacute
weakness

categories of, 41
definition of, 41
West Nile virus (WNV), 12, 78, 155
WNV. *See* West Nile virus

X-linked bulbospinal muscular
atrophy, 155